Suicide Junkie

by

S.Westwood

Published by:

Chipmunkapublishing

PO Box 6872

Brentwood

Essex

CM13 1ZT

United Kingdom

http://www.chipmunkapublishing.com

For Ashley 'You and me vs the world'

The Nails In My Coffin

Dear diary.

I am thirty-one and have the scars to prove it. I might look young in face but in heart and soul I am truly ancient. I would have been ready to pack this all in years ago but my persistent breathing is a habit I can't seem to break. It's not through lack of trying, but here I am. I long for cancer, to be diagnosed terminal. That would be so perfect; to be able to die without the stigma of suicide, to know that I haven't got long to endure. To have all those people caring about me. 'It's such a shame, you are so young.' And I would have to act all down trodden and sad when inside I would be laughing. I could pick out my own coffin and plot of land where I choose to be buried. I could organise which songs I want at my funeral. Tori Amos 'Tear In Your Hand' and the Smiths 'I know it's over'.

Writing here is the only way I can show the world how I really feel without actually killing myself. I can't bear to think that I am a nothing, that I have nothing to show for being in this hollow world- so I write in the vain hope that something will come from it. And all I know and have to write about is my feelings of utter despair.

Only I know how awful it is to live with these feelings, with the wish to not be here. I am lacking what makes me the human animal I am supposed to be; I am lacking the instinct of survival. I feel that I have always got this choice to make and when I wake up in the morning afraid that I have to live another day, it starts to influence my decision. The temptation is too great. I constantly think about it, constantly looking for a way to make it better, or a way to make it end. Like having a song playing constantly in your head, the only way to get it out is to play the damned thing. There is only one way to stop thinking about suicide, and that is to do it. I want to do it. I want to be the one that the system failed. I want to be the one that actually does it, not just someone that talks about it all the time. I want to have the power of my convictions. I want to show them all. Prove to them. Give them something to think about. If I could die by will alone I would have already spent about thirteen years in my burial bed.

...But here I am. I go to therapy, I take the pills. I sit with the psychologist tapping my face and body, saying those words 'I completely accept myself'. Well yes, I do accept it. I accept that I am depressed, that I hate myself and hate living in my mind, that I hate the world and want no part of it. I accept that there is no grand reason why we are here. I know that there is no meaning or purpose to any of it and therapy is not going to change that. I am intelligent. I am introspective. I am a writer. I have the ability to see things for what they truly are and you only have to read a paper or watch the news to see that humanity is an abomination. I know there is no truth in religion and I hate the damage that it does in the world. We made it all up to try and explain this planet, this life that will never be explained. How can all the religions be right and if a single one of them is true, then what sort of God is he? How can God let us live like this? Don't get me wrong; I would love to believe in something. To die and to not even know that you are free of this place is a scary prospect. I want there to be an afterlife. Sometimes nature enthrals me so much that it seems impossible that there is not some grand creator, other times I am trapped in a secular hell.

My hatred for everything or my total apathy about it all is the hardest thing to live with. I have no energy, no get up and go, no ambition. When I lose all hope that things might change I see no point in stringing this out. I sometimes have things to look forward to, things that I hold on for, yet when they come I do not feel the pleasure in the way that other people do. I have lost the ability to 'enjoy'. I am an ingrate and it doesn't matter how wonderful my life becomes it will still be 'life' and I still won't want it. I could win the lottery and I would still be miserable. Hope that things will ever be better seems like stupidity or blind optimism. If your glass is half full you have probably drunk so much of it that you no longer care. Mine is completely empty.

Yet I live. I live and I write in my diary about how I feel, unable to tell another living soul. No one wants to hear it. No one wants to be confronted with someone that wants to die. It is my dark secret. The fact that I am not planning to live, but I do try to live. I try to act normally. It's like there are two Stephens inside of me, one that wants a normal life, and one that wants me dead. It is a constant battle that rages in my head that no one really knows about. I am alone in this, trying to convince everyone, including myself, that I am going to have a full and long life while the other me, is shaking death by the hand.

Am I completely selfish? Is that what all this is about? I must be because the one thing that scares me more than living, more than death, is surviving another suicide attempt. Then I would have to face up to my actions. Then I would have to try and mend the relationships that my selfishness has destroyed. So why do it? Why do I have such strong suicidal urges? Why have I had these urges all these years? Why does it seem to bear no relation to what is actually going on in my life? Why won't the God damn shrinks tell me that one? Have I got too much of the suicidal gene in my DNA? Are there too many suicidal chemicals in my brain? Can't they give me a pill that deals with that? They can't can they? They send me to therapy with three different people and not one of them has been able to touch on just why. Why a kid from the country village of Wymondley grew up from catching newts and making camps to slashing his wrists and taking overdoses. Surely there is something in between those two events that has made me this way?... But no one can help me and I have always been meant to kill myself, so that's what will have to happen. It is my unwritten destiny. It gets to the point where I feel that I really have to do it. It is not even a choice anymore. I must obey.

You might ask how I can do it to my family. How I can do this to the girl I love. Well, the guilt I feel about my plans to die is just as strong as my urge to carry them out. It is as if someone else, the other me, made those plans me. When Ashley comes home from work I usually put that other me aside and I am there for her, but sometimes he stays like a great dark cloud smothering my thoughts. Living for the sake of someone else is not easy. I wish that I wanted to live for myself, but I probably never will. Have I chosen life by being with Ashley? I keep putting off my death but in doing so I am just putting off my life. Sometimes I think that my death would be for the best. I am a burden and will be a greater one if time goes on. I am better in spirit than in flesh. The memory of me would be much more pure than the real Stephen, and I need something pure. Well the only pure thing in life is death. I should quit while I'm ahead. I am nothing but a worry to my father and mother. I am a misery to friends and others. I am someone they just wish was different. They wish I was well. Well I'm not, I won't ever be and don't want to be. I want to have never been born. Failing that, there is only suicide.'

The First Attempts

My childhood was not bad on the face of things. I was not abused. I was not neglected. Our family was not particularly impoverished, though certainly not well off. I remember many things fondly and still love many of those things that the child Stephen held dear. I may have grown out of wanting to be a cowboy but there are films I went to see at the cinema when I was a child that I have since bought on DVD and watch regularly. I think that is true for a lot of people. What we loved as a child shapes our personality and you can definitely tell what sort of person someone is simply by whether they do or do not like 'Labyrinth'. Why should we, as 'grown ups' lose the magic of innocence? Many of us still hold on to those feelings and by watching those films or listening to the music we grew up with we can recall those chaste emotions. Things look better in a mask of nostalgia. I may have cried and been taken out of the cinema when I watched Star Wars for the first time but at least I can boast that I saw all three films of the holy trilogy on the big screen. Adam Ant may have lost his looks and gone a little insane, but he will always be cool to me and the Muppet show will always be the most perfect family entertainment.

Babies are born with eyes about 75% the size they will eventually be in adulthood and that's why they look so disproportional. I was born with huge crystal blue eyes and they are my most distinct feature to this day. Girls tend to say that they are attractive where as guys think they are plain weird and that I should blink more often; I am a 'guy'. My white blond hair grew out to brown and has since been dyed black. I have tried to stay away from my natural hair colour for a good fourteen years. I haven't been well for longer…but I was a baby once with all his life ahead of him, beauty on his side, so what went wrong? It must have been something in my upbringing. There must have been something while I was growing up that changed this trouble free child into the wreck I became, but it's nothing obvious. We have to delve deep.

I was the second child. My sister Jane is four years my senior. I was born as her play thing. I was born so that I could be a companion for her. Is that not why people have more than one child? I guess most kids are born out of selfish reasons. I was not asked whether I wanted to be born and I know why babies cry. When they slapped me into life it was taken as a personal insult, but was I already the person I was going to be? How much of it is down to our genes and how much is taught? Twins grow up to be individuals despite having the same upbringing and the same biological make up. What the hell is it that makes us, us? Why the hell did I become so messed up?

There was nothing in the first few years that could possibly be to blame. My mother was still married to my father and my grandparents were alive on both sides of the family. Admittedly my parents should never have been together but I doubt that I could see it at such a young age. I remember going on holidays with both parents. I remember my dad making a sand sculpture of a speed boat and remember him saving me when I nearly fell down the side of a hill and down through someone's thatched roof. That was my first brush with death. Perhaps I liked it.

…But I was a happy kid as far as I know. I got on with my sister, most of the time. There was one occasion when she strangled me against the wall until I went purple but I don't hold that against her. I have looked through the photographs of me as a child and I seem perfectly happy in all of them. I suppose pictures are not the best evidence though. People don't take photographs of pain, of unhappiness, of disappointment. There are photographs of my birthdays taking new toys out of their colourful wrappings. A bendy Kermit the frog, a big blue car, a weeble circus. Of course I am smiling in all of them. You get told to smile even if you really don't want to. Those toys are almost gone from memory now and would probably be gone completely if it wasn't for the photographs. If only I still had them I could make a fortune on eBay. …But we tend to not remember much from our early years. I often wonder though, when we are toddlers, do we remember being babies? As babies do we remember being in the womb? Why is it that all of that is lost? Why has it all become a mystery when we all go through it? It seems that to forget must mean that it was not important, yet that is not true. If you are abused in your early years the affects, if not the memories, fuck you up for life.

Well, I was not abused. I was looked after, bought presents, baked cakes, taken on holidays. I was a normal kid. The only thing that might be a factor in my downslide is the relationship between my mother and father. It was rocky. There were arguments. I don't even know what the arguments were about but I remember them yelling at each other. I would lie in bed listening to the theme music of M*A*S*H and then the shouting would begin. I think they actually booked themselves in for a nine thirty argument each night. They probably thought that I would be asleep but their yelling was a nightly lullaby for me. Did I know that they did not love each other? Did I suspect that daddy would soon be leaving us? They split up and the arguments ended.

I grew up in a small village and there was plenty of countryside all around us. I had a whole world to explore. I would spend my days wandering around the fields, making camps in the trees and wading through ponds in my wellington boots. Sometimes my sister would be with me, other times I was all alone, but I never minded that. There was a lot for a child with my imagination to do and I was content to spend my days alone with my mind. On reflection that was probably not for the best. Too much time thinking means you think about too many things. I guess when my father left I spent a lot of time thinking about that.

11

I loved trees and climbed most of them in the village. If I couldn't get up one then it became a tempting challenge. I used rope to try and get up, I ripped my jeans scrambling up the trunks and then there were the ponds; I loved them too. Over the field that we called 'Beware of the bull' due to the old sign post by the stiles were two areas, which were always filled with water in spring and summer. The ponds, I was told, were formed in what was once the moat of an ancient castle. There was nothing of the castle left, if indeed there ever was one, but the moat appeared to be there all the same. I would spend hours looking in those ponds catching newts and frogs and then putting them all back before going home for tea. Once I caught so many that I think I must have emptied the pond. I had about one hundred of them in a bucket waiting to be put back. I still have a soft spot for newts; they are a much underrated creature, but not very good at avoiding nets. I remember the smell of those ponds, stagnant water and wet dirt and cow shit, why then do I remember it so fondly? I was a boy; I guess that's why. The world was all new to me and there were adventures to be had. Once I crossed a muddy patch in the fields and I was not quick enough and sank in the black wet dirt. I was stuck there, literally, and my sister was trying to pull me out. Eventually she pulled me free but my boots were left behind enclosed in the muck. My mother was not too pleased.

Sometimes I would embark upon what I thought was a grand expedition. There were thickets of trees in the middle of the farmed fields and I wanted to investigate them all. I would set my sights on one distant wood and decide that it was about due an exploration. I would pack a bag of reserves and take with me a strong stick that would be my walking cane and sword. Off I would go, looking for signs that the wood was a home to monsters or used for witches' black mass rituals. I would sometimes find overwhelming evidence! Some of those wooded areas were very creepy and my sister would tell me stories about them. I found a dead bird hanging by its legs on a fence post once and there seemed to be no innocent explanation for it. There was another pond fifteen minutes walk across 'Beware of the bull' that we called 'Stocking's pond'. Apparently a horse had broken its leg there and drowned. For some reason I found that very spooky and very sad. Then there was the thicket of trees we called 'The spinny'. There was a pond in there that we always kept a distance from as we were told that it was bottomless. I believed it all.

Kids are very gullible and you should be careful what you tell them. There was a large hole in my grandfather's nose just by his eye and I obviously asked him where it had come from. For years I believed him when he told me that a frog had bitten his nose. Truth was that he had cancer and, although they had removed a tumour, he soon died from it. My dad's dad was the first death I had known. I think that even came before my first hamster. I was never that close to him but that didn't make it much easier. I felt guilty that I didn't feel bad enough about it. I didn't know if my reaction was wrong. I didn't know how I was supposed to act. I didn't know if I was still allowed to smile. I went to the funeral but couldn't help enjoying the melancholy of it all. I liked the seriousness. I liked the shinny black hearses and the flowers. I liked the fact that we were supposed to be sad, that we had all congregated in that place for the purpose of sadness, and then there was the finger food that came hours later. It was a party for sadness! I found that I was quite good at being sad.

Perhaps I have got into the habit of being miserable. Perhaps I find it easier. Perhaps that is my natural state of being. When I was a kid my mouth used to be open, that was its natural way, yet I trained it to shut as I grew up. Perhaps we have to train ourselves to be happy. Perhaps I just haven't got the energy to smile. Perhaps I'm just too lazy.

I began to display a morbid curiosity, a penchant for darkness. I liked horror stories and read 'The Little Vampire' books, which tapped into something in my mind that would never leave. Another haunt of mine was the church yard. I knew my way around there well. I had taken etchings of the tombstones and read them all wondering how that person had died and seeing how old they were. It seemed all the better if they had died young but there were very few young deaths in that graveyard. I had searched the whole church yard looking for the vampire vault, but had come to terms with the fact that my graveyard just didn't have one. I was very disappointed.

One day I discovered a forgotten grave that was so overgrown with grass and weeds that it was completely hidden. It even had a fully grown tree growing in the middle of it, its roots probably smashing through the coffin below. I was disgusted that this person had been forgotten and I spent a whole day clearing the weeds and cutting the grass. I worked hard and was sweating and dirty by the time I had finished but I felt that I had done a truly good thing. No doubt the weeds soon grew back, but at least I had proved that this person was not completely abandoned. If the spirit of that person still lingered on Earth then he was sure to be pleased. That may well be the one act that sends me to heaven, the most altruistic thing I have ever done.

...But do I believe in heaven? Heaven and hell are a Christian concept invented to make us all tow the line. Better be good or you'll go to hell and what happens to suicides? It is throwing God's gift of life back in his face, that must be a ticket to Hades. People used to believe that a suicide would become a vampire, or would be trapped on Earth forever as a ghost. That was, unfortunately, all in the past.

I did a puppet show once about heaven and hell. I think that is quite important to realise that, even at such a young age, I thought about those things. I don't remember the script but I know that it was a love story between an angel and a demon. I had quite a lot of puppets but Monkey

Doo was my favourite. That monkey was almost surgically attached to my arm for a good few years. I had a whole world created for him and he was a theatre, movie and singing star. He was getting so worn through use that I asked for a new one at Christmas to replace him. Of course I was far too in love with him by then to get rid of him, he was still my favourite and he got married to the new monkey that I named Monkle. I still have both of them, I always will; they are lying together in my bedroom.

Give something a face and it instantly has feelings. You can't throw away your old teddy bears or puppet monkeys because they are alive! If they have a face then they can think and feel. I still find it hard to eat ginger bread men or jelly babies.

I spent a lot of time writing and practicing my puppet shows. I was enthralled by the Muppets and also tried to learn ventriloquism from books I ordered and took out of the public library. I think I got quite good at it and I know that I should have followed my ambitions. I could be working for Jim Henson's company by now puppeteering or using animatronics on new movies. That was where my life would have gone if only I had faith in myself. Being depressed makes you feel that you are no good at anything and that you have nothing to offer the world. I think I have got nowhere in life because I have no skills, the truth is that I have got nowhere because I think I have no skills. I can't imagine myself being able to do anything. I don't drive, not solely because I am afraid of it, but because it is something that other people can do. What other people can do, I cannot. I wait in the queue at the post office and watch the people working there and I think 'how can they remember how to do all these different things, I couldn't do that. 'I buy something in a shop with my card and I think 'I don't know how to take money from someone's card'. Everything that I don't know how to do adds a link to the chains of self-depreciation. Yet these are simple things, and I am not an idiot. Yet I sometimes think I am, sometimes I think that I know and can do nothing.

I have always needed to have little projects on the go at all times, and I have dipped my finger into all sorts of pies. If it wasn't my puppet shows it was writing my children's book about Harry the hedgehog. If it wasnot writing it was programming my Spectrum computer. If it wasn't that it was building board games. I had to create, and I still do it to this day. As I got older I saw where my skills lied and decided that I was a writer. What I am writing now is my latest venture, but it is hard to have hope. Sending off samples of my books is like pulling the plaster from an injury that has not yet healed, exposing it to the elements. When all the replies come back negatively it is like salt rubbed into the wound. So many times I have lost all hope. So many times I have tried to come to terms with the fact that I am just this, a nothing who will never be published, who will never be anything. I'm obviously just not good enough, but I need it so bad. I need to create. I need to write. Only when I'm writing do I feel I have any worth, even though I'm usually writing about having none. Yet why bother if no one is going to read them? Why bother if this is all just a pipe dream? Perhaps I will be famous when I'm dead and they will make documentaries about me and put out a page spread in the daily newspaper. Perhaps my life will gain cult status. Perhaps I will just be forgotten.

Recently I have fallen out with just about everybody in my family, but when I was young I really looked up to my sister. She went to the same school as me and I was always trying to hang out with her and her friends. I suppose that it must have been really annoying for her but if she ever showed it I didn't notice. I had friends of my own of course, but she was always my best friend and we spent a lot of time together. She would come with me over the fields with one of our neighbours that was the same age as her. I tagged a long. There were other kids living near by and they would sometimes hang around with us. It was such a small village that we all knew each other. They were all nearer to my sister's age so I was always the youngest and, I guess, Jane's unwelcome shadow.

I had a few friends that are now so gone that I don't even know if they are still alive. They could be in prison; they could be high-class lawyers, I just don't know. No one I knew from primary school went to my secondary school and the friends I once had were friends of a different person. They had been friends with a child, and I was not him anymore. I would have liked the purity of only ever having the same friends throughout my life, just as I wish that Ashley was my first and only love. Life is not like that. My life is a mess of people coming and going.

I had always striven for purity. I have always been ashamed of my weaknesses, of my animalistic humanity. I have always wanted to be beautiful and innocent. I have always wanted to be kind and good like an angel. Where I got such ideas I will never know. My family is not religious and I have never believed in any of that. I have made my own morals and I have tried to stick to them but just where they come from is as great a mystery as the origins to my depression. Perhaps those things were taught to me, however subtly. Perhaps I learnt it all by not learning anything.

I learnt things from the older people I hung around with, though now in retrospect, nothing useful. They were people to look up to. I liked being around my sister and those other slightly older people. They talked about things we weren't allowed to talk about…but did I want to be more grown up like them? I guess I did. I guess every child wants to be older. If only we were young with an adult soul, then we could enjoy the beauty and freedom that children have. Youth, as they say, is wasted on the young, but being young was the only time in my life that I did not feel the weight of the world, the weight of life, resting on my shoulders. It was all spoilt by the wish to grow up. Did I feel that I was older

17

than I was? Did I feel that I had to grow up faster and be the 'man of the house'? That was something that the early trips to the psychiatrist seemed to suggest and when was the first time that I went to see a shrink? I have to admit that I don't completely remember. My memory is useless. Things are forgotten to make room for new things to forget. I don't remember the exact time that it all went wrong. I don't know when the puppet shows ended and gave way to fits of tears. I don't recall the downslide, just a number of events that marked what was going to be my life to come.

When my parents separated I had to make the choice of who I would be living with. How can a child make such a decision? I think it was always an unwritten agreement that I would live with my mother. I don't think my father even wanted me. Every Sunday he would come around to see me and take me out. It must have been hard for him only seeing me for that short time and not knowing what to do with me. I was nothing like my father. The main difference being that I did not like sport and that was all he had to offer me. We sat in the car watching a local football match and I sat uncomfortably bored until they finished. Then he drove me back. His main interest was lawn bowling and I eventually took an interest in it so that I had some way of connecting with him. For a while I played the game and got fairly good at it. My attention span, however, kind of drifted.

I may not like sport but I am more like my father now than I realised or wanted to admit. My mother had poisoned my mind against him. She said he was a pig, a chauvinist. She said how he was a typical man as if that was the worst thing to be. She told me that a lot of their arguments had been about how he would shout at Jane and I and the names he used to call me. I had it drummed in to my head that I should not be anything like him, that I should try not to be a 'man'. Here were my first lessons in growing up with an all female household. This was my first realisation that I could not be what I strived to be.

Then my sister was taken ill. She had woken up one morning with knees like footballs. She ached and she was losing weight. She was becoming so thin that she looked like she was being starved. I didn't know what was going on with her and she was getting a lot more attention from my mother, being taken to hospital appointments, having tests and seeing specialists. She was given plaster casts that she had to put on her legs when she slept. She ate dinner with us and then threw it back up onto the plate. My mother was getting angry with her and with the doctors because they didn't know what was wrong with her and she just didn't know what to do. My mother was at her wits end.

Apparently, I attempted to jump out of my bedroom window. I can actually remember being there, on the window ledge with the window wide open looking down at the ground and wondering if I would die if I jumped. Perhaps it was just curiosity, perhaps I didn't really want to be dead, but that is probably just wishful thinking. The fact is that I did it. I was a kid and I was thinking about suicide. At sometime my mother must have come into the room and dragged me away from the window, God knows what she must have been thinking. She got what I was trying to do out of me and the next thing I remember is being at the child psychiatrist in London, being asked why I would want to jump out of my window. I laughed because it sounded so silly, because the man sounded so terribly serious. I guess even then my attitude towards death was quite flippant. I didn't have much to say to the shrink. I was a kid after all. How could a kid explain something like that? I just didn't want my life anymore.

That was the first time. That was when darkness came into my life. That is when the idea occurred to me that I did not have to go through with this; that there was a choice to be made. I think that is my main problem, the fact that I see it as a choice. That I can choose having a wife, going to work, having children, or I can choose not to choose life, that I can choose to die, right now. We are all going to die one day but why wait? Why do we bother going through this hell just to end up at that same fatal point? Let's speed up the process. Let's decide how it will happen. No more waiting for the inevitable violence that is dying. No more bringing people into your life just so they can be destroyed by your passing. No more years of life that makes the dying even more difficult to get away with. Let's just do it, let me do it, let me die.

Most people don't have that choice to make. To most people suicide is not even an option. They have problems and wonder how they are going to get out of them, but they don't think 'never mind I could always just die'. I have been in the company of people and heard them mention suicide, but to them it is a joke. They say 'this is music to slit your wrists to', unaware of the times that the blade has travelled across my flesh. Unaware that I have listened to those songs over and over while I watch the blood congeal on my arms. They say 'I may as well just kill myself' yet the actual eventuality of doing it is never further from their minds. They make jokes about it without for a second; stopping to think that there might be someone listening that is really affected by the issue. It makes me recoil with unease. I hate people making light of it, belittling the way I feel. 'Cheer up it might never happen', well what if it already has?

I started to get ill. I remember the pains in my belly and they were excruciating. I remember my mother driving me to school and I was in the back with the pains. I needed the toilet and I was trying to keep my mind off of it by singing the song from a peanut butter advert over and over in my head, over and over so that it was irritating the hell out of me. Along with that, was that other voice in my head that had started to come all the more often, that mocking whisper 'yeah, yeah, yeah...' That journey was a little slice of hell. I couldn't tell my mother I felt ill, not now she was driving towards the school. I had to bear it, those minutes that felt like hours, each bump in the road making me feel sick.

When we finally reached the school I stood outside in the cold with a friend, the pain not ceasing, until I plucked up the courage to ask a teacher to let me in to the toilet. I could literally feel the colour draining from my face. The teacher took one look at me and let me pass.

That was the last day I went to school for the next three months. My mother was called to pick me up as I was complaining of a sore belly and because I had been sick. I hadn't been sick at all, but I knew that if I told them that they would have to send me home. I spent the rest of the day lying on our sofa with a blanket over my body. In the 'comfort zone'. ...Home where nothing bad could happen, home where I could be looked after.

My sister was still ill, but I was ill too. I was having these pains and I could not go to school. I would cry because the pains were so bad, doubled up on the sofa. The doctor had been called out to the house because I refused to go out but he could find nothing wrong with me. Yet I felt just awful. This went on for a few weeks and I maintained that I felt too ill to go to school. The doctors said it was probably just a virus or whatever excuse they could find for their incompetence, but the truth was they just didn't know. I have never really thought about how dreadful this all must have been for my mother. Here were both of her children, ill with mystery illnesses; she must have been tearing her hair out.

Eventually they decided that there was only one thing that could be wrong with me and that was appendicitis. I still had an appendix and my pains were, apparently, somewhat similar. They would have to do tests. I frightened my mother so much with my screaming and crying that she got me admitted to hospital. That was not an unknown place to me; my sister had been there a lot. We used to visit her and I would sit writing stories while my mother tried to make my sister feel more comfortable with encouraging words and gifts. Jane looked so ill it was frightening. She was so thin

21

that you could see the bones in her face. There were tubes in her hand that attached to a drip beside her. I don't know what I made of it all; I didn't know that my sister would have only had two weeks to live had they not admitted her in time.

I hated being in hospital and was a terrible patient. I hated being woken so early, hearing noises that made me think I was at home until I opened my eyes and found myself on that horrible sterile ward. I hated all the tests and I hated the food. I refused to eat and the nurses force-fed me. A nurse spoon-fed me corn flakes and the milk was cold. My mother always gave me warm milk with my corn flakes. I spat them out into the nurse's face.

I don't know how long I was there, not long I guess. I had all the tests and they came back negative. There was nothing wrong with my appendix. There was, they said, nothing wrong with me. Yet still I had the pains and still I felt the sickness. I refused to go back to school feeling so terrible. When my mother tried to make me go I cried the house down. I screamed and held my belly saying how sore it still was. I went to the toilet and stuck my fingers down my throat so that I threw up on the floor. Seeing that convinced her to keep me home. I expect she felt guilty for doubting me.

I guess it was a hard time for my mother having doctors say there was nothing wrong when there was obviously something not right with her son. There had to be an explanation. What was really wrong with me? What had started all of this? I spent days and days lying on that sofa feeling ill and feeling scared while doctors refused to admit that there was anything the matter. The truth was that I would do anything to keep myself from going back to school, and although I wasn't purposely faking an illness, the illness was, never the less, fake.

22

Soon enough the stomach aches weren't needed anymore and they went away as miraculously as they had arrived, but I simply would not go to school and if it was ever a possibility that I should go back, I started crying and throwing a fit. I don't know what was making me so unhappy. I did have friends at the school. I was not being bullied. I was not finding the work too difficult. I just couldn't stand the thought of being there. Of being taken out of my comfort zone. Of having to face all those people for all those hours. I just didn't want to go to school. You can hardly blame me. When you are that young all you want is your family, your mother, yet they make you spend hours away from them every day. It's a wonder we don't all go insane. Well, my mother thought that I might be mad and she took me to a local shrink. There I was asked loads of questions that I did not want to answer. How I felt now that my dad had gone and what was it like growing up in a house full of females. Looking back at it and thinking about how I am now, those questions were really quite valid. Growing up with my mother and my sister meant that my main role models were female and they were teaching me to not be like them. I didn't have my father's opinions on things and the older I grew the less we met. No wonder I ended up hating men and striving to not be one. No wonder I sometimes wished that I was female.

I truly have gone through stages in my life where I wished I could change gender. I have always looked up to females and their lives and thought that they were so much more attractive than men. Not only did I find them more attractive but I also wanted to be that attractive. I have never been homosexual, but perhaps I could be a gay female? Then I could make my face up and wear cool clothes and just be utterly gorgeous. Then I wouldn't be a man, an animal, an impure pig. Perhaps I am exaggerating, for I have never actually felt that I was female, just wished that I was. I prefer the way they live; I prefer the feminine position in life. I am in touch with my feminine side to the

23

point that I despise my masculinity. This is due, no doubt, to my upbringing.

My sister left the school we both went to and started 'big school'. She would come home and tell me stories about the naughty things she and her friends had got up to and I looked up to her thinking how totally 'cool' it all seemed. We still had a good relationship but she wasn't spending as much time with me as she used to. She would spend a lot of her time in her room listening to music. My love for music started around that time and in those early days what my sister liked- I liked. When she liked Madness and Adam Ant I liked them too. Now she had begun to listen to heavy metal and it all seemed so grown up. I wanted to like it too and soon began to get into the bands that she had already grown out of.

'Big school' seemed so much more interesting than anything I had known, a whole other world. When my sister allowed me to be with her I felt that I was part of it and talking to her made me feel more grown up myself. She sang me the songs that she had made up about her teachers and she told me how she had drunk 100% volume alcohol in her chemistry class. Even talking about doing chemistry sounded so much better than what I had to do at school. Perhaps I would be better once I started secondary education. Perhaps the only reason I hated school so much was that I had already grown out of it.

My sister showed me some little blue stones that she had stolen from the chemistry lab and she told me that they were highly poisonous. I held them in my palm staring down at them. That royal blue colour certainly didn't look natural and I had no reason to doubt what she had told me. I had never seen anything like them before. As she wrapped them back up in tissue paper and put them in a tin, I was already making my decisions. She put the tin away in her bedside cabinet.

She went to school the next day and when I thought the coast was clear I let myself into her bedroom. Her bedroom was very pink, as mine was very blue. The wallpaper was light pink and her bed covers also. Scattered around were old soft toys and a doll that I remember as an icon of the eighties - a white clown with black spots on its clothes. I looked in her box of cassette tapes, at the Iron maiden albums that each had the same monster on the front cover painted in different surroundings. I had heard that the band were Satan worshippers and I wanted to be one too. There were supposedly hidden lyrics in some of the songs that you could only hear if you played the track backwards. I wondered if my sister had those albums and whether she had heard those lyrics. I liked the darkness that those heavy metal albums seemed to portray. I liked the front covers with their monsters, skeletons and graveyards. I liked the danger and the rebelliousness. I liked the thought of immersing myself in that world, but what I wanted more was the very reason I had come into my sister's room in the first place. I wanted to die and she had the method there in her bedroom, she had those blue stones.

I opened the bedside cupboard and surveyed what I saw. The tin with the stones in was sitting on top of some books in the bottom part of the cupboard. In the top part were lots of magazine clippings and bits of scribbled on paper. There was a musty but pleasant smell that I knew to be the incense sticks that were in their packet and shoved between two books. I took the tin and sat on the bed. I opened it and put the lid to one side. There were the three little tissue wrapped packages. Slowly I unwrapped one and sat there looking at the blue stone in my hand. It certainly did look as though it might be poisonous, just like my sister had said. So, with the belief that this could kill me, I put the stone in my mouth and swallowed it whole.

I waited all day for death to take me, for something to happen. I lay downstairs on the sofa where I had spent many weeks, waiting. Evening came and my sister came home and all I could do was worry that she would find the stone gone and tell my mother. Nothing was happening to me. I had a slight stomach ache but even the stress of what I had done could have caused that. I did not feel the excruciating muscle contractions of a slow acting poison. I did not feel sleepiness over coming me that could have slowed my heart and made it stop and when I went to bed that night, it seemed painfully apparent that I would, in fact, wake up.

I still went to the shrink but I never told him about that incident. I never told him how bitterly disappointed I was to still be living. I had made an attempt to end my life, an attempt that had taken courage and despair yet here I was talking to this man, this stranger, about life. Perhaps he helped. It was so long ago that I don't really remember what we spoke about or what his answers were. All I know was that I went, I talked, and eventually I was well enough to go back to school.

I remember that first day back, unsure how I was supposed to behave. I felt normal, I felt well and I don't even remember feeling particularly anxious yet here I was going back to school after three months of therapy and pain. I didn't know if I was supposed to act as though I was still ill. I didn't know if I was supposed to fool all the teachers into thinking I was still frail. Well I didn't fool anyone. I teamed back up with my former friend as though everything was perfectly normal. Neither of us seemed to mind that we had not seen each other for months and he never even asked me why I had been away. We played and chased each other and to get to him I jumped over a table and slid along its surface. A teacher saw me do it and shouted at me. I stood there scared of being told off and the teacher said, "You seem to be completely better don't you?" It was said accusingly and without sympathy. I had let down my pretence and I felt bad that now the teachers would think there was nothing wrong with me at all. However, there was something wrong, and it wouldn't be long before it emerged in a different guise.

·

The Prelude to Prozac

The first two years at secondary school were not too bad. No dramas, the promise of a decent education, the excitement of learning new subjects and finding new friends. I was not bullied or disliked. Why then did I grow such a desperate hatred for myself? It was a gradual decline.

I had started to delve deeper into my dark world and I was slowly uncovering more and more darkness to envelop myself in. My only father figure was my mother's father and I was taking up a few of his hobbies. My granddad loved horror. He liked the old black and white Universal monster films and the Hammer Horrors from the sixties that they sometimes put on TV after midnight. We didn't have a video recorder but I was sometimes allowed to stay up late at my granddad's house watching those movies. I loved them, especially the vampire ones. There seemed to be such a haunting romance to Dracula, a man that looked human yet was so much more. A man who was attractive to females yet had a dark secret. I wanted to be him; I wanted to be a vampire. I read Dracula, which was a hard book to read at that age, and I borrowed others from my granddad getting further and more deeply involved with that dark atmosphere. Once I had read Anne Rice's 'Interview with the vampire' there was no turning back.

I wrote my own vampire stories playing out my fantasies, that wish to be like them becoming more and more pervasive. I rushed home at night to watch the TV series of 'The Little Vampire', a show that showed a young vampire making friends with a mortal. I so wanted that to be me, for a vampire to befriend me so I could persuade it to make me a vampire also. I wanted to be able to fly and see in the dark. I wanted to sleep in a coffin and hang around the graveyard. Everything I did was about vampires; every book I read or film I watched. Every English essay and class talk. Told to make up a story about a pet, I chose a bat. Told to speak to the class about something from history, I chose Vlad the Impaler. It got to the point that my teachers were worried about me and called my mother into the school. The English teacher told my mother that everything I wrote was about vampires or some other horror and my mother asked whether the essays were well written. That soon put the teacher in her place. They couldn't say that my work was badly written; I enjoyed English most of all and always had a flare for it. Faced with that fact my mother said that she had no worries and the teacher was left floundering.

Halloween was a favourite time and I always had a little party up in my loft which was above my own bedroom and which my father had carpeted and given boarded walls. My sister and I used to do it, just her, her friend and me, but she was older by then so it was just down to me now. I invited a couple of friends over and we dressed up and played spook related games like apple bobbing and pass the parcel with a ghoulish prize. I remember dressing up as Beetlejuice and feeling quite disappointed at my friend's attempt, which was just a few scars stuck to his face. It seemed that only I felt that Halloween was important. I would be better off living in America around that time of the year, and if I hung about there a while longer I could muscle in on thanks giving as well.

I still don't know to this day if the loft in my mum's house is haunted. I guess it was just my sister or mother trying to make Halloween more exciting for me but there were some strange goings on every year. Things would go missing, like my sister's slipper. We looked everywhere in the loft for that bloody thing. We even tipped out the box of magazines and comics and looked all through them. It was not in the loft where she had left it so we searched the whole house. I found it eventually. It was placed under the top magazine in the box in the loft, the place we had looked for it already, and then there were the lights. We would leave the

29

light on in the loft, go downstairs for something and when we came back up the light was off. It was strange, yet not quite evidence. I sometimes wish that something supernatural would happen to me just so that I can have proof of the after life, but I don't know if I could handle the experience.

Some of our traits must be passed to us genetically. The fact that I liked horror and monsters so much had to come from my granddad. The fact that I liked to write, even in my spare time, must have come from my mother. I never thought I had much of my father in me, but then I didn't know my father that well. Now that I am older I can see ways in which we are similar despite the glaring ways that I am different. Some of it is genetics and some of it is learnt behaviour. I don't know where I got the insanity from, where I got this desperation but I was becoming the person I was going to be. Darkness was both my friend and my enemy.

I think in the first couple of years at secondary school you are all still kids and can all get along with each other; it's when you become teenagers that things get nasty. I was doomed to become an outsider when adolescence hit. My love of darkness and my delicate sensibilities were bound to have me ostracized. Not to mention that my hair was now getting quite long and I liked heavy metal music. If you are not like everyone else your life is going to be hell and that is an accurate description of my early teenage years.

No one wanted anything to do with Stephen Westwood, not even my former friends. Luckily I had found a constant companion in David, a kid as equally impaired as me. Together we would get through it. David would prove to be my friend throughout the rest of my school days and without him I might not have been able to cope.

If I had wanted to be friends with the others I guess I could have changed. I could have listened to their music, cut my hair, been less individual, but I stuck to my guns no matter how hard that was. I didn't pretend to be anything I wasn't and didn't hide what I was. Yet every week it got worse and the jibes and taunts took their toll. It didn't seem to matter if these people knew me, if they were in my year or in my class, it seemed to be a conspiracy with the whole school to make my life miserable. I was called ugly, I had endless comments about my hair and my eyes, and I was pushed around. Those things matter, even though I hated those kids as much as they hated me, being hated takes it out of you.

The bullying was always just a step away from physical. Things were called out across the playground as we walked from one school building to the next. 'Greebo' was a derogatory word that apparently meant someone that likes rock music. That was my name to all that didn't know me, and to those that did it was still my name. Either that or the sarcastic taunts of 'nice hair'. Then of course there were the 'uglys' and the 'wankers' and all the other general swearing. They also made it hard for me to relax in class. Things would be thrown at me; my things were stolen from my desk and thrown around the classroom. I was constantly on guard because they always made it clear that they were going to do something. I always feared that they would spit chewing gum in my hair, and that did in fact happen a couple of times. Basically, I was shown complete contempt, no respect whatsoever. I was shit to them and enough abuse like that and your self worth goes right down hill. I began to hate myself as much as everyone hated me.

It was even worse for David. I was, for some reason, one ounce better than he was. He would get pushed around where, as I would only get threats. One day three of the main bullies grabbed David and proceeded to try putting a condom over his head. They just wanted to belittle him as much as possible, to take away all of his dignity. I was afraid of those boys, they were much bigger than I was but I wasn't going to let them do that to my friend. I stepped in and together we fended them off. For an hour or so we were respected for sticking up for ourselves, then that was forgotten and we became dirt once more.

By the time I entered the third year I had become paranoid about my looks and personality. When I get paranoid it is not just a simple delusion of persecution, it is an all-encompassing phobia. I began to get obsessed with my cheeks and nose that I was convinced were red. I was paranoid about spots, although I never had acne and never thought badly of anyone that did. I just couldn't cope with my skin being anything but perfect. All those years of being a child with pure skin and now I was hitting adolescence and my face was changing. I wasn't pure anymore. I would spend all day at school afraid that someone would notice and pick fun at me. When they said I was ugly I wanted to crawl into a deep hole and hide away. It's true that even to this day I do not know if I had a real skin problem or not, all I know was that it was real to me and I couldn't bear it. I wanted to hide. I didn't want anyone to see me. I stared into the mirror and I cried, hitting my head against the glass. I wanted the pale perfect complexion of a vampire. I wanted to be beautiful and it seemed so unfair that I had to put up with my looks being so inferior.

So one morning when I was feeling particularly bad, I raided my mother's make up case and found that she had foundation cream. I knew that it could be used for covering what you didn't want people to see. I knew that it could be used for covering blemishes, spots and redness. When my mother wore it her skin looked perfect. It was my only hope. Rushing to get ready for school I covered my face in the stuff and left to catch the bus. My paranoia that day was building like a dark storm cloud in my mind. I spent the day in fear, my mind never leaving the thoughts that were focused on my skin condition. I thought that everyone was looking at me, examining me, talking about me. All eyes were looking at Steve, all laughs were about him. The whole school was talking about the fact that 'Westwood' was wearing make up.

It wasn't right for a boy to be wearing foundation cream, no matter how much better I thought that it made me look, and I feared the reprisals if someone saw it. I had put it on to try and make myself feel better about how I looked but I didn't feel better and I knew that I would not be spared a beating if one of the bullies noticed. Wasn't it better to have bad skin than to wear make up? I just wanted to hide the real me, I wanted to have control over how I looked. I didn't want to accept that I was ugly, but all day I thought about nothing else and thought that I must truly look like a freak.

At every opportunity I was in the toilets checking my face in the mirror. It looked as bad as I thought. The make up was overly brown and didn't match my normal skin colour. My nose had little flakes of skin visible because the make up was caught up in it. I looked monstrous in my eyes, deformed, my face peeling away to reveal a creature inside. I wanted to wash it all off and start again yet I wouldn't dare to remove the make up now. I didn't want to see what was underneath and I didn't want anyone else to see. I knew my face would be red if I washed it and I had no way of covering it back up. I wished that I could run away, out of the school and back home. Yet I stayed all day, and somehow I got through it. No one at school had ever said anything about my skin in the past and no one, in truth, said anything now. It was as though there was no difference and no one seemed to notice that I was wearing foundation cream despite the fact that it was applied by an amateur in a rush. I had got away with it.

Things got worse rather than better. Finding a way to hide my skin soon became a necessity and I became a prisoner of my own disorder. Every morning I would rush through my paper round and get back home to the bathroom mirror to apply my mask. The paranoia never left me. I got better at it yet it didn't matter how good I made myself look it was never good enough for the rest of the school. I was still called names, was still persecuted. I worked hard to make the make up look natural, to hide the skin but to also hide the make up. I must have been quite good at it for never in the whole of my school life was I ever taunted for wearing make up. No one noticed, but they hated me anyway. Even David didn't notice and if it was helping me get through school, then why did it matter? Well it did matter. It mattered that I was afraid of the rain, afraid of the gym showers, afraid of sweating or rubbing my face in fear that my mask would slip. It mattered that I couldn't just get up, comb my hair and go to school like everyone else.

I stared at the other pupils, examining their skin. Was I the only one? Did any of the other boys wear make up? Some had perfect skin and it made me sick with jealousy. Some had spots yet none looked as bad as me. If I got a spot it would dominate my entire face, sending it out of proportion, ruining the symmetry. When the other boys got spots they just looked like an unwelcome addition to their face, it didn't entirely change what they looked like. I had it worse than anyone. I was disgusting.

That problem began at school and only got worse with time. I hated my face and hated that I had to show it every day. I pulled my hair down over my eye as if it would hide me, but I was never hidden enough. I spent hours on my skin each morning yet still I was taunted, called ugly and shown only contempt. I know that my continuing lack of self esteem was all due to those names they called me and the constant harassment. I know now that a lot of my later problems came from being ridiculed at such a young age. Those things can really stick. My hatred for the vast majority of the human race comes from spending my school days with complete arse holes.

...But my life was not just school. Out side of that my life was better. David lived close to another boy, Rick, who went to a different school and who we both became friends with. He also liked heavy metal music, was growing his hair and was getting picked on. We were three misfits

34

who stuck together and saw it through. When we were together all of that stuff didn't matter anymore, we had some good times, and we laughed a lot. We were very good at generally mucking around and amusing ourselves. We watched 'Bill and Ted's Excellent Adventure' while drinking beer and reciting the script. I don't know how we managed to get the alcohol because none of us looked old enough for that. I guess we had just found an off license that was happy to make its money even if that was by selling booze to underage teenagers. If we couldn't get beers, Dave had a great habit of raiding his parents' spirits bar. He would get a cola bottle and fill it with a lethal concoction of spirits and bring it over to my house. Most of the time it tasted foul but we drunk it anyway. Sometimes Dave would bring one of his cocktails to school and we would drink it in our lunch break hiding in an underpass. Once we had to do a sponsored walk around Stevenage and Dave and I were very drunk by the end of that! We had found a way to feel good, and drink was that way.

Dave, Rick and I spent the vast majority of the time drunk. We looked for other ways to make ourselves feel good and experimented in a number of ways. We tried cigarettes but they weren't great. We made roll ups of many of the things in my house and tried smoking them. We smoked tealeaves and mixed herbs and a crushed up cigar. We took painkillers with our drink to heighten the experience. When we weren't drinking, and I guess, sometimes when we were, we played in our punk band Revelation. We all wanted to play music and so we each bought an instrument and thus a band was born! Dave bought a guitar, Rick bought a bass and my drum kit was an electric Yamaha affair with touch sensitive pads that had to be plugged in to an amp. Luckily for us we had an amp as my mums' latest boyfriend had left it at our house and my mother had dumped him.

My mum had a string of loser boyfriends that either left her after one night or fucked her up over a period of time.

She and my sister would go out together to the Red Hart pub where they were known for getting drunk, chatting to the 'lads' and dancing on tables. I can't think of anything worse to be known for. Every weekend they would go out and I would stay home, sometimes with my mates, sometimes alone, and await their return. I didn't know what to expect when they got in. I didn't know what state they would be in or who they were going to bring back with them. I would lie in bed and hear their staggered heels on the path outside my window listening to their slurred voices and listening for the sound of a man. Quite often there was a man, sometimes two, sometimes more. My mother would come in to my bedroom and invite me to come downstairs to 'smoke' with them. This was what I had to learn from. I guess allowing me to do it was better than having to do it behind her back. Truth is, I never much cared for it as it often made me feel sick.

I can analyse reasons why I might feel the way I do about things in life. I know that the hell I was put through at school destroyed my self esteem and I know that seeing my mother with all those blokes gave me a twisted, although not completely untrue, representation of the male species. They were there for a good time, to drink, take drugs and get laid. My mother and sister probably knew that and knew what they were doing but in my eyes it was wrong and they were being used. I think that I had nothing to rebel against and rebelled in an opposite direction. I swore to myself that I would not be like those men, just as I had sworn that I would not be like my father. The only man that held any redeeming features was my grandfather, and I clung to that role model, putting him on a pedestal he could never hope to live up to.

Dave and Rick thought my mother was great, and I guess I liked the fact that I could get away with so much. I was allowed to drink and smoke and stay out late or over night. I could go to Bowes Lion and watch live bands, get drunk and then sleep on Dave's bedroom floor. We put on a Revelation show at the village hall and bribed people to come. It was basically just Dave and Rick's friends. They each got a bottle of thunderbird wine for coming, just so that we would have an audience for our one night only gig. We were terrible and none of us could play but we enjoyed playing music together, writing songs about drinking, girls and how stupid people who liked hip hop were. We played our songs to these few people as they got drunk and we got drunk as we played. I still have the tapes we made as that band including some of the live tracks we played that night. It was a laugh. Everyone was drunk and throwing up outside the hall. Rick went into the kitchens and bent all the cutlery. 'Drunken youths' were apparently seen roaming around the village. We were subsequently banned from ever hiring the hall again. We thought that was very cool.

None of us had girlfriends and the girls at school hated us, but that was something I did want in my life. There was something lacking and I presumed that a girlfriend was what I was missing. Dave and Rick were good fun to be with but I craved love. I never chatted up girls when I went out. Most of the time I was too drunk to even think about approaching anyone, but mainly it was due to my low self-esteem. I would spend hours getting ready to go out, putting on my make up, foundation and eye shadow. I didn't try to disguise the fact that I was wearing make up when I went for a night out but made it part of my persona. Everyone accepted that I wore it and looked good for it, though I was still very insecure about my looks. I was still putting on a mask and I hid behind it, like the phantom of the opera, and no one would be allowed to get close enough to me to unveil the real Steve. I felt doomed to never have anyone get to know me in case my changing face would one day let me down.

It's hard to explain, for while I did look in the mirror and think how good I had managed to make myself look, even though Rick, for one, would say I looked great, I never believed that I would actually be attractive to the opposite sex. The hatred I seemed to inspire in the girls at school

37

made me wary of ever attempting to find anyone out side of it, but I wanted it so bad that I put an advert in Kerrang, a heavy metal magazine, asking for female pen pals. I guess it was obvious that what I was really looking for was a date, but it worked. I got a lot of replies. I guess the photo of me, taken from a good enough distance to make my skin look fresh and clear, had fooled them. Perhaps once they met me it would be different, but for now I was just planning to write back to some of them and see what happened. I wrote to some that were not local but who sounded nice and shared some of my musical tastes. I also wrote to Anne who was from a village not too far away. We spoke for a while through letters and then we decided to meet up. It felt like a real 'fuck you' to the people at school. My life outside of that hell hole was fine and that was what was important for me to hold on to. Outside of school, with the people I actually chose to   mix with, I was perfectly popular.

I met Anne at the Stevenage rail way station and she was with two other girls who were introduced to me as Winona and Erica. I knew that she was bringing these friends with her and didn't mind as it made things a little easier for me. What if there was a lull in conversation? Well that shouldn't happen now that there were others there. They were all alternative looking girls and I liked the look of all of them.

Anne had light ginger hair and a long face. As I was attuned to noticing such things I noted that she wore a lot of make up. Winona was a little plumper in the face though not at all fat. I don't think she was wearing any make up. I noticed she had very pouted and full lips. Erica was the oldest and seemed too mature for me. They all wore simple t-shirts and jeans but I already knew that they were all heavy metal fans; I knew we had that in common.

We walked around the town together talking about the things we liked and things we had done. I didn't try to be anyone I wasn't but kept up with the conversations. I would guess that I came across as quite shy for I wasn't used to being in that kind of situation. I was with good-looking girls, all of who were single and all of who would be making judgments about my personality as the day went on. It sounds like a nightmare actually. I got through it though. We did a bit of shopping and I made them laugh a few times. I didn't really know what I had to offer them but it seemed that laughs were one thing I could give. I was more out going in those days, with the vitality of youth. I just allowed myself to act a little crazy and they seemed to like that. Anne and I swapped phone numbers before we got on separate trains home. I was excited, not really concerned as to whether I liked them but simply concerned that I had made a good impression. Were they feeling the same? Were they trying all the time to be someone I would like and so concerned with that that they didn't actually notice me? If that was the case we both had nothing to worry about did we? No one was noticing anything!

I phoned Anne a few days later and she invited me to come to her house. I had begun to ride a scooter and was, therefore, able to ride to her village the following weekend. It was quite a distance actually and I was thankful that I had this mode of transport. It would give me some independence and would allow me to start a relationship with Anne. I guess I was jumping the gun a bit. I was sure that we were going to be boy and girlfriend. At her house I was allowed to be in her bedroom with her and we played music and talked a while. Then it came to pass that we were both lying on the bed and we hugged each other, her head on my chest. We lay like that for an hour. I was excited, wanting to take it further, to kiss her, to 'make out', to have my first experience with the opposite sex. Nothing else happened. I went to kiss her and she turned away. Maybe that was moving too fast. I had no idea how to act in such a situation. Maybe she was not ready. She was a year younger than me so perhaps girls of her age didn't kiss boys. I was naive and didn't know what I was doing. Or was it that she just didn't fancy me that she had seen through my disguise and was repulsed by my skin? I felt exposed and uneasy; I wanted to get to a mirror quick. But instead I left. The hug was nice, it was a start.

Anne phoned me a few days later and said that she didn't want to go out with me again but that her friend Winona liked me. She gave me Winona's phone number. I didn't know how to feel. I was cut up that my first brush with a girl had ended so abruptly but I had not become that attached to her yet and I was being offered another chance. We vowed to still be friends and would no doubt see each other again (Winona lived in the same village as Anne) but there would not be anything romantic between us. It was strange. I felt hollow, excited, and afraid. I called Winona.

Winona was pleased to hear from me but tried to act nonchalant. She had obviously told Anne to give me her number but now pretended that she didn't expect the call. It was a fairly easy phone call despite the fact that I usually hated speaking on the phone. I asked her if she would like to come to my house and she said that she would. Her parents brought her and I met her at the bottom of the road, outside of the pub, so that they didn't get lost looking for the house.

I felt great as I saw her step out of the car and come towards me. Here was my first girlfriend and we had the whole night to chat and get to know more about each other. It is so exciting when you first meet someone that you are attracted to. You want to know everything about them and can't wait to find it all out. And I honestly believe that if you have had that first moment of attraction then that will stay and nothing that they say or do will shake it off. I was attracted to Winona and that was that. She shouldn't have been worried as to whether I would like her, for I liked her already. I guess that's what is meant by love at first sight, simply that your first impression sticks. Getting to know the object of your attraction and finding out things that are good about them is just a bonus.

We walked up to my house and we held hands straight away. There was a chemical reaction in my brain and in my body the moment we touched, teenage adrenaline. I really didn't want to blow it now, but I had a strong belief that I wouldn't. I felt empowered by the vibes that she was giving off. She liked me, it was obvious. She didn't think that I had bad skin. She didn't think that I was stupid. She really liked me.

Winona did become my first girlfriend. At the end of that evening I walked her back down to the bottom of the road and there, in the dark and in the shadows we kissed. It felt wonderful, felt exciting, felt like a beginning. I had crossed the line between child and man. I was a teenager and would enjoy it.

The kiss was not executed brilliantly but it was ok for the first time. Our teeth knocked once, but we didn't stop. At length her father's car came to a stop on the other side of the road and we stepped out of the shadows and said our good-byes. I couldn't wait till I saw her again. I had been accepted.

The next time I saw her was when my mother and her male friend arranged that we should all go and see a band in Bedford. That was not rare. Quite often we would all go out as a group to see bands and my mother would lie to the bar staff saying that I was 18. 'I should know- I gave birth to him!' I don't know how we got away with it.

We picked Winona up in my mother's car and we both sat in the back. My sister was going to meet us there and she would come with her boyfriend by motorbike. Winona's parents must have been very trusting. They had no idea what they were allowing their daughter to do. I guess that with my mother there they felt it was fine- well they hadn't met my mother had they? There would be much drinking, much trouble making. We were out for a good time.

Our mouths were busy that night and we didn't care that we were in public. I think that I was the first guy she had kissed and she was the first girl and we were just enjoying the new experience. I imagine that it was quite embarrassing but I didn't feel it. The band was one I had seen a few times before and had actually got to know a little. My mum and her friend were not shy and would often chat to the band before and after they played. The members of the band were happy for me that I had found myself a girlfriend and teased me in a friendly way. I felt extremely grown up and I think Winona looked up to me as I was older than her and had this whole life. I had this to offer her- good times, drink and bands and kissing and everything else. She had no idea how naive I really was.

We were boy and girlfriend and we hung out together in her village along with Anne sometimes and other times we went out with her and her other friend, Erica, who always seemed to like me a little too much. None of them disliked me because of my skin. None of them knew I wore make up, but one day we were in the tennis courts having a game and it was hot. With the heat of the sun and the exertion of the game I was sweating and I was getting very paranoid about what I looked like. I knew the make up would be running and I imagined drips of brown liquid rolling from my nose. After the game Anne laughed at me, pointed and said, "You've got sun burnt on your nose! How embarrassing", and it was. The redness of my nose had been noticed. It wasn't just in my head any more it was there in fact. I was mortified.

I would still see my friends. I was still the same person I had always been and still wanted to get drunk with Dave and Rick. Winona couldn't come with me but didn't mind me going to those weekly 'piss ups'. The thing was though; something else had been introduced to me and was taking over from my love of alcohol. LSD was now becoming my drug of choice and we would do it every weekend. We would take it and go for walks around Stevenage in the middle of the night where the streets and houses suddenly became interesting and new. The roads were like soft beds that we rolled on. The trees moved and breathed. Everything was in soft focus and so much more beautiful. When on that I felt so happy, content and free. I felt like a gorgeous vampire prince out in the night where I belonged. It may not be an addictive drug but the need for it was there all the same. It changed my world and I only wanted the one that was induced by that hallucinating drug. It didn't matter that I was coming down during lessons at school. It didn't matter that my mother was against doing anything as strong as that and would have been upset to find out. It didn't matter that I kept it from Winona. It was mine and I embraced it.

We would have parties where we did nothing but talk all night, from seven till seven, laughing and pointing and telling each other how the drugs were affecting us. "Look at the lampshade man", "watch the carpet and see the patterns swimming". We listened to the same music over and over, listening to it change every time, never getting bored. Then I would go home and go to bed telling my mother that I had not been able to sleep all night because it was uncomfortable on Dave's floor. I would lay in bed for a few hours playing games on my Sega, getting totally absorbed in it as though it were all real and then I would sleep for the rest of the day.

I was coming to the end of my school life and was taking exams but that was the last thing I wanted to think about. My mind was full of Winona, drugs and drink. I was having the time of my life and didn't want to have to think about work and studies. I was still getting abused at school but my life outside of it was so much more important that I could laugh off all the taunting. Out side of school I had a girlfriend and a life. I wouldn't let them grind me down any more.

Once someone pushed me while I was doing up my shoelace and I fell forward hitting my nose against the wall. It gave me a cut and it made me see red. People saw how angry I was and were urging me on to punch the guy. They were laughing and shouting. Then one of the bullies grabbed him and held him and said "come on Westwood, hit him". I wasn't going to do it- not like that, but the anger was like burning fuel inside my chest. The teacher opened the door and called us in for the lesson breaking up the commotion that was centred around me. I said that I would get him after the lesson was over and I knew they would hold me to that.

I couldn't concentrate on my studies for the next hour and a half; I was just worried about the fight that I was going to have, worried that I would fail, that I would get hurt. I had never been in a fight before and the whole thing didn't sit right with me. I was not the sort of person to throw his weight around like that, but there was part of me that had just snapped. It's one thing to call me names but I had always decided, in the back of my mind, that if ever it got physical I would fight back. Part of me realised that if I saw fury I could be a vicious little bastard. Part of me just wanted to get a little respect and I knew that in that school using your fists was about the only way to gain it.

After the lesson I waited for him by the door and when he started to come out, he saw me, and went back in. So he was scared of me was he? That felt weird, I liked it. I ran to the other doors and when he came out of them I didn't stop to think. I didn't think about all those dreams I used to have about punching people with no effect. How I used to have no strength. I didn't think about my worst nightmare that was to get my nose broken, making me uglier than I already felt. I didn't really think about getting hit at all, only about hitting him. I punched him twice with my right fist and once with my left and then he ran away. There were cheers and laughter and for a day I was looked at in a different light. I wasn't someone you could just abuse. Steve would take no more shit.

People still made fun of Dave and me but it would soon be over. Both of us were planning to leave school after the exams and real life could not be as harsh as this. We drank in our free periods and Dave would often take the whole day off. People called us 'alchees' and 'druggies' but they didn't know the half of it. I was drunk in my biology exam and passed with a D.

I met Winona when she finished school, standing there by my scooter sipping beer from a can. I thought I was so grown up, so revered. I had finished school; she had another year to go. Our relationship had blossomed into puppy love and we experimented with our sexuality in a very immature way. We had not gone all the way yet, but we had both said that we wanted to. The truth was that I didn't really want to. I just thought that I was supposed to. That's what you do when you love someone isn't it and losing your virginity is supposed to be so important, such a step on towards adulthood. Perhaps I still wanted to be a child. I don't really know the main reason but I was scared to death of the whole idea. There seemed to be so much pressure. It had to be at the right time, in the right place with the right atmosphere. Winona's parents had to be out. Well it wasn't long before that time came.

Everything was in place. We had the house to ourselves. We had protection. We had the music on the stereo. We were kissing and taking off our clothes. We were lying together and getting ready to do it and I tried to make the right moves but... She just lay there, naked and ready for me to do whatever it was men were supposed to do, but I was nervous, petrified more likely and she was just, well, laying there. The whole thing just stopped, failed, retracted like a child touching the eyes of a snail, it was a total disaster. I felt sick, I felt cheated, I felt like I wanted the bed to suck me in and spit me out at my own house. I wanted to hide and not speak about it again. From that second on my hatred for the whole act was set in stone. I didn't want to try again and I didn't think I would ever do it; I didn't think that I was capable. I didn't want anything more to do with sex and give it a week or so and Winona didn't want anything more to do with me. She dumped me for a guy even older than I was. He was a guy that no doubt took her virginity- a task that I had failed so badly at. A lovely moment turned to complete embarrassment. I wasn't so grown up after all.

The break up of my first real relationship hit me hard, even more so because I felt that it was my sexual disaster that had turned her off me. It began a six-month routine of mourning, drinking and taking LSD to try and forget. I had begun college, which I was only doing because I had failed my math's GCSE, but I had no passion for it. I just went through the motions not really participating in the experience. I was not ridiculed at college though; I was accepted and had made a few friends to speak with in lessons. Here my alternative look was just one of many. There were others like me; there were people that dressed even stranger. Every day I wore the clothes that I always wore out side of school, and no one paid me any mind. I wore my Megadeth T-shirt and my tight black jeans and instead of hurling abuse they tried to get to know me. Could one year make so much difference to maturity? Or did I just go to the most fucked up school ever?

The new friends I had made noticed how down I was and they were concerned, but I knew what I needed. I needed to get drunk and I needed to be with Dave and Rick with a tab on my tongue. I span out of control. LSD heightens your feelings, and I was depressed. I remember one night I smashed a glass on the floor and stuck my hand in it, shaking it around until I saw a good stream of blood. I ran out into the street, running across the roads without looking out for cars. I was inviting death but it would not come. I had to live with the pain of rejection, the pain of failure and the pain of loss. Thankfully getting wasted does make the grieving go a little smoother. Time, however, proved to be the greatest healer.

And so I went to college and I did my work and I was free of the horrors of school. The teachers treated me like an adult. The pupils treated me like a human being. If I felt too down to go in there would not be any questioning or punishment. If I wanted to talk there were people there that wanted to listen. I was fairly popular, though I always thought that the girls looked at me as if I was a weirdo. Perhaps they did. I wore black clothes and had long brown hair. My fingernails were long and sharpened to a point. I made no secret of my love for dark things, and that love was only getting deeper. My bedroom at home was painted dark grey and black with vampire movie posters, fake cobwebs and plastic bats hanging from the ceiling. I was a gothic monster made by my own design and I was sure that I was quite unattractive to 'normal' girls, but I was pretty much done with the opposite sex. My life was girlfriend free, partly by my own choice and partly due to the feeling that I had nothing to offer anybody. I had seen Erica a few times but I only ever saw her as a friend and despite the obvious fact that she liked me I was done with relationships.

I concentrated on other things. I had bought a real drum kit and was teaching myself to play. I joined a college band and we practiced on Sundays. I kept my previous friends and we still got stoned and drunk at every opportunity. I went to see bands in London, taking LSD and gliding around the tube stations like I was some supernatural entity. I went to parties and had chances with girls but I actually remember turning them down by saying "I don't do sex" and "Sorry, I can't, I'm depressed." Everyone thought I was weird and I guess I seemed quite content to be so, but there was no real contentment. I was at complete odds with my sexuality and the person I was. I had created myself, but I hated him. I was a secret to myself and a stranger to everyone else. People thought they knew me, but my persona was a mask, just like my make up, and I hid behind them both.

I dyed my hair black and began to dress more like a Goth than a heavy metal fan. My music tastes while always centred around rock, were becoming broader and darker. Punk was always there, as something I really went for and I wanted to play in a dark punk band rather than the indie college band that I had ended up in. I was learning from it though, learning to be a better drummer, learning to write songs, learning social skills with these people that I wasn't very close to but that I was spending time with. It wasn't long, however, before I told them that I was leaving the band and they were very unhappy with me. I remember that Dave, Rick and I decided to do acid over at my house during one sunny day in June, as my mother was on holiday. We were running around my garden pointing at flowers when the whole of my estranged indie band turn up at the house wanting to 'discus' my decision. It was the most surreal experience ever but when they realised I was completely out of it, they left well alone and they did not try and get me back again. I think I scared them away. I realised that I was, in fact, quite scary.

I guess I was getting more and more uncomfortable with myself. After college I was on the unemployment line with no ambition. The only thing I liked was music but I didn't really expect or even want to get famous as a drummer. I had got my math's GCSE but I didn't know what I wanted to do next. The future was a scary prospect and I was out in a world that I felt too fragile to be in. It seemed that I had a hang up about everything; about sex, about my face, about my personality. I was a waster, a drunk, a druggy, a lazy loser.

I quit taking the drugs in the hope that I could regain some purity yet the only time I ever felt pure was when I was stoned. I wore the make up twenty four seven and would not even let my mother see me without it. I went out less and stayed at home all day trying to find things to occupy my brain. But with so much time alone, all I could think about was me and how damned depressed I was. I lay in my dark room with the curtains drawn and prayed that a vampire would come and take me out of the boredom that was human life.

I started a band up with Rick and a girl he was friends with who played guitar. I focused all of my energies to that, spending my days writing songs and making posters. It was my baby and it gave my creative urges something to focus on. They would come round and practice in our dinning room that had become the constant home for my drum kit. My mother was a good sport; I guess she knew how important it was to me. We called ourselves 'The Fiends' and we played punk music in the style that I had always wanted to play. I wrote songs based around the Hammer Horror movies that I so loved and that I now collected on video. I had over a hundred vampire movies in my collection and they were all I ever watched. I dressed and acted like a vampire myself and became 'vampire Steve' to everyone that knew me. I went to see bands at the weekends and sometimes our band would play. We would get drunk and have parties. I should have been happy, but a dark cloud hovered above my head all the time. A dark cloud I had got so used to that I didn't even take an umbrella anymore, but my life would have to change. I couldn't be a teenager forever.

At length I found a job. I became a hospital porter. At first it made me feel grown up, made me feel like I had moved on in my life, but I didn't do very well for long.

This was because the paranoia that I had over my looks, increased ten fold. I was constantly in view to the other members of staff, the patients and the public. All those eyes were looking at my bad skin, at my spots, at the redness, at the make up. I felt that I was always on show and I was always thinking about it. Some days I would be in the bathroom trying to get ready for work and it just wouldn't go right. I would cover my face in make up, work on it for an hour, and then wash it all off and start again. When I washed it off I always looked worse than I had to begin with and I didn't know if I could make it right again. Many days I would be sorting my face out until the time came that I would be due to leave for work, and I would panic because I hadn't finished. Some times I would go in to work half ready, thinking about how awful I must look and hiding from jobs in the toilets. Other times I simply couldn't leave for work and I would finish sorting my face out and turn up late. Other times it would just be useless and I would not go in at all.

Every morning was the same. Get up and run into the bathroom before my mother could see me, and then force myself to look into the mirror. I always hoped that today would be different, that today I would look ok, but that day never came. I would wash my face and pat it dry with the towel, sometimes I would bury my head in it feeling safe that my face was completely hidden, wishing there was a way to feel like that all the time. It wouldn't have mattered if it were my legs that were bad. If it was somewhere like my legs it could be covered up and I could lead a relatively normal life. But this was my face, constantly on show, with only make up to aid me.

I had got used to the ritual but I hated going through it. Applying moisturising cream and then the foundation from my mums make up box. If I applied it as cream it was too thin and you could still see what I looked like underneath. So I used the slightly thicker cream that had congealed on the underside of the lid, scraping it up onto my nail and smoothing it over my nose and over my cheeks. I would blend it in, trying to make it look natural, and then I would take the small stand-alone mirror with its magnifying glass and look at each little area of my face to see if I had missed anything. My face changed depending on which mirror I used and how close to the daylight I stood. I hated looking at myself in daylight. I tried to avoid it completely.

I remember one particularly bad day I was trying to get my face sorted and I couldn't and I was sitting on the bathroom floor crying into the mirror. I did the best I could but you could see that I was wearing make up. The redness of my nose had been greater that day and I had needed more layers yet my skin was a little dry and the make up was showing. The redness hadn't gone, the make up was showing and I had a spotty area under my chin that just wouldn't cover up. I looked like a freak. I tried and tried. I washed all the make up off and tried again, doing everything the way I always did yet this day it just wasn't working, this day I just looked too bad. The panic was growing inside of me, my hands were shaking and I couldn't keep the mirror still. A huge lump had formed in my chest like I had swallowed a boulder and couldn't digest it. I dropped the mirror and started crying pitifully, pleading with whatever God was listening, to please make my skin ok. The time was ticking. I kept looking at my watch but there just wasn't time to make it right, to pick off all the dry skin, to blend in all the make up. I sank down with my knees drawn up to my chest and I cried still pleading, "please make it stop".

I sat there watching the time on my watch go past the time that I should be at work knowing all the while that I wasn't going to make it. I felt physically sick and was shaking all over. I didn't want to look at myself anymore and now that I knew I wasn't going to make it in to work the stress lifted a little. Eventually I left the bathroom that I had been in for over an hour and I phoned in sick. The boss was mad at me, telling me that I had a responsibility and that I had done this too many times, but how I could I be seen today? How could I let the other staff members and the general public see this monster? I went back into the bathroom, washed off all the make up and started again.

It took another two hours in the bathroom before I could go out, and the only reason I made myself leave at all was that I was getting truly scared of myself. I walked from my house in Wymondley village, four miles across country to reach my mother's work in Letchworth. I just wanted to be with her, I wanted a cuddle, and I wanted to be told it was all ok. I trudged over fields and then back on the road and eventually, after hours of trekking, I reached her and I hugged her and I cried, but nothing had changed. Things were far from ok.

I was depressed. The job wasn't helping. Slowly but surely my employers were getting fed up with my unreliability. I was called in to the office and told that I had to smile more, that I had to talk to the patients and make friends with the staff. I was told off for being so miserable and I was told off for my constant lateness and sickness. They had no idea that there was something really wrong with me and I didn't really know it either, except this couldn't be normal. Other people couldn't feel like I do and get on with their work. I was mentally incapable of doing the job. I was mentally incapable of leading a normal life.

I worked in the old people's wards and there I saw the putrid decline of human existence and there I saw death. I would have to wheel the old people into therapy and sometimes I would have to pick up a body bag from one of the wards and take it to the mortuary. I thought that was kind of cool, but it couldn't of helped my state of mind. The wards smelt of old people, of soiled sheets and unwashed flesh. They were there waiting to die, and I saw it all.

I hadn't known much death in my own life. My dad's dad had died when I was young but it hadn't really affected me. What affected me now was my other grandfather's admission into the hospital where I worked. He was close to dying in the intensive care ward as I carried out my duties elsewhere. When I had my breaks I would go up and see him. I wanted to talk to him but I felt stupid. He was sedated and he didn't even know I was there. I whispered to him and I told him how bad I felt. I told him things that I could tell no one else. I told him that I wished it were me that was dying. I told him that he just had to get better because I loved him and he was so important to me. And all the while, I felt bad because there was one strange and little part of me that welcomed the misery. The fact that I had a real reason to be sad made it easier for me to be the way that I was. I had an excuse and if he were to die, I could be miserable forever.

At length he got a little better and was moved on to a normal ward. I think he had heart disease although I never really understood what was happening to him. He had not had a heart attack or a stroke, he was just slowly dying. He wanted to go home, and after a time they let him. It was obvious that he wasn't well, yet there he was in his white vest walking up his garden path inspecting his roses. He wanted to be at home to die. No one was saying it but that was what was happening. He bought us all a little present and it killed me to take it. He bought me a book called 'Lazlo Count Dracula'. This would be the last thing he could give me. Any day it could happen. All the time we were on edge that these could be his last moments. He wasn't home long before his condition deteriorated badly and he had to go back to hospital.

I lay in bed and by candle light I read the book my granddad had bought me. I was about half way through it. I spent so much time in my darkened room watching vampire movies and reading vampire novels that my brain was filled with gothic darkness. It wasn't miserable to me. It was the way I was and I had to be comfortable with it. The thing was though; it meant that I could not function in everyday life. I was attempting to live as a human being but I did not fit in to their world. I was an outcast. I was useless.

As I read, the candle began to flicker and dipped so much that shadows cloaked the walls and I looked up from the book and looked towards my door. I had a feeling, a strong and definite feeling that my granddad was there, but that was impossible. He was ill in hospital and my mother was at my grandmother's house to keep her company. I was alone yet I definitely didn't feel that I was the only one there. It could mean one thing and one thing only, my granddad had died and his ghost had come to see me on his way to the next world. I was sure of it, the feeling getting stronger and stronger, and I stared at the door in fear that it would start to move. I said in my mind over and over "please don't show yourself it would frighten me" and soon the candle stopped flickering and the feeling left me.

When the phone rang early the next morning I knew exactly who it was and what they had to tell me. It was my mother and she said, "I have some bad news." And I said, "I know, granddad is dead", and he was.

I remember his funeral. I cried as I watched his coffin slide behind the curtain. It was so final. He was really gone and here was a funeral, something dark and gothic, yet there was no pleasure in it, not even for 'vampire Steve'. This was the end of my grandfather. For all of his strange ways he had still been like a father to me at times, the only constant father figure I had, and now he was gone. I hated that he was being cremated, for that was like utterly erasing him from the world, but his ashes were buried in Hitchin cemetery and I would visit him there sometimes. I would take a few beers and sit with him while I drunk them, chatting to him quietly about how bad I felt, about how I hated my job and hated my life. He was the only one I told, it was my secret and I felt that I had no choice but to just get on with it. ...But there had to be another way, this was so hard.

Life went on and left me behind. I was terribly depressed. I felt like I had fallen into a deep dark pit and there was no means of escape. Darkness surrounded me and I wallowed in it alone in my misery. No one really knew how I felt. I was terribly lonely. I would seclude myself from my mother and from whatever boyfriend she had at the time. I would stay in my dark room and watch my horror movies on an old black and white TV. I would drink cider and eat popcorn though I ate little else. I had begun to worry about my body as well as my face and would try to keep a count of the calories I consumed every day. I would try and eat only one thousand calories a day; an amount I now know was terribly low. I had no reason to think that I had any problem with my weight as everyone thought I was skinny, but I wanted to be. I wanted to be slim and pale and beautiful. I weight trained for an hour every night even though I hated it. I hated the exertion, the sweat that washed off my make up. I hated doing anything other than lying on my bed. I turned down nights out because it would interfere with my routine and because I wanted to be alone. I saw less and less of my friends though somehow we kept the band going and I focused on that as much as I could...But it was going nowhere really and I needed something to change. This half-life just couldn't go on. Spending all of my time worrying about how I looked, panicking in the mornings and hiding when I got home. This was no kind of life.

Then, I lost my job. I remember how it felt. I had worked a whole shift, I had worked bloody hard and then they asked to see me in the office. I sat there feeling terribly small with my two immediate bosses staring at me with an unreadable, serious expression on their faces. "Stephen, we are making cut backs in the porters section and we have decided to let you go...starting immediately." I was dumb struck. I was being sacked and for what reason...because I had never quite 'fitted in', because I wasn't 'jolly' and 'chatty'. I was being sacked because I was bloody depressed! There was nothing I could do or say to change this. It had happened. I had been sacked from my first job; rejected. I was just not good enough.

My depression just got worse and worse. Now I didn't even have work to get up for. I spent entire days in my bedroom so that I didn't have to go through the bathroom ritual.   I spent all my time worrying about how I looked and keeping away from everybody.   All day I was alone, my mother was at work, and all day I would be aware of every boring depressing hour that went past.   I drank pints of water and starved myself eating nothing but a few slices of bread and feeling guilty about even that.   I weight trained in my room each night hoping that it would keep my body from deteriorating though never wanting to grow muscle.   I quit the band and stopped going out.   There was nothing in my life now.   Something had to give.

I went to Stevenage and I wandered the town, my brain enveloped in darkness, my mind trying to make a final decision.   I went into Woolworths and tried to look around but there were so many people.   Their faces seemed to grow and to come nearer to me, distorted and grotesque.   They were all looking at me.   They were pushing me, getting in my way, so many of them all breathing my air and I could not get a breath.   I panicked.   I looked all around me, and those people were everywhere.   I began to sweat and my heart was racing.   I had to get out.

Once outside I felt a little less claustrophobic.   The panic attack lessened a little but I had to get further away, I had to be alone.

I went to the shopping centre and got in a lift to the top floor.   There I stood on the balcony and looked down to the shops and the shoppers.   Everyone was going on with their stupid little lives.   Everyone was oblivious to me, to my terrible anguish.   Well if I jumped they would be aware of me wouldn't they?   ...If my body came falling down, smashed and bloody on the tiles, then they would notice.   My chest was tight and my stomach was still churning.   As I looked down, the ground seemed to spiral away from me, or to come closer.   I could not judge the distance or decide whether it was high enough to kill me and I wanted to die.

That's what I had decided. I didn't want to live this life any longer.

I didn't think it was high enough so I walked to the top of the multi storey car park and went straight to the edge. I looked down. It was high, high enough I imagined although I had no way of knowing for sure. My body was still going through a panic attack, my breath coming in spasms. I didn't have the guts to do this, to actually jump. It was so harsh, so frightening. Yet it seemed so easy, just one step, but it is so against human nature that I didn't think it was possible. Christ how bad did I have to feel before I could get up the courage to kill myself?

I turned away from the edge and took one deep breath. This wasn't going to happen, not today.

I went in to the public toilets feeling terrible, feeling my depression weighing me down, feeling physically sick, and shaking with nerves. I looked in the mirror, gripping the sink with both hands staring at myself, staring through my reflection and looking at the soul within. The soul was broken, the mind was mush. I breathed heavily and I kept on staring despite the strange looks I was getting from a few men that came and went. I didn't know how long I was standing there before a security guard came in.

"What's wrong with you?" He said.

Leave me alone, why can't I just be left alone.

The guard went behind me and checked the cubicles. I stayed in the same position watching him in the mirror.

"Are you taking drugs?"

"No. I'm fine." and I had to be fine didn't I? I had to try and act normal despite the fact that I was mentally ill. I had to get another job and I had to live a life. If I couldn't kill myself, then I was trapped here. If I was too damned chicken to put an end to the pain of living then living was all I could do.

Bring back Erica into the equation.

She had been at university and had just finished the year. She, who I had always known liked me, gave me a call and asked if I would like to go to the cinema with her. It was an unexpected offer and my mind looked for reasons to turn it down, but why should I? My life needed something fresh and there were definitely no other flames on the horizon. I was at a loss, at a loose end and this seemed to help tie it up. I agreed to go.

We met at the cinema. I was dressed in the way I had adopted, tight   black jeans, pointed gothic boots and a white vampirism poet shirt. I was wearing a lot of make up and my hair was long, black and covered one eye. My mother always said that I would lose the sight of my eye if I wasn't careful but I ignored her, and I was right for I can still see perfectly fine. Erica hadn't changed. She was thin and looked as mature as always. Her hair was brown with a hint of red. As I got closer to her I began to think that she was fairly pretty, although I had never been interested in her before. I wondered whether it was because I was older now. I wondered if Winona had been too young for me. I wondered what this friendly meeting might turn out to be.

We went for a drink first to catch up. We talked a lot as we had done a lot of things since we last met up. We had both been through college and she was going back again after the holidays. I asked her about her studies, we spoke about music, a subject I was still passionate about. I made her laugh telling her about the indie band I had been in, about the fact that it really didn't suit me and that we had even had a saxophone player! She spoke about her ambitions, about her family, her student parties. There were no awkward silences. I liked her. I had always liked her but something was different now. Perhaps I had grown up?

We went to see 'Natural Born Killers' and I was quite excited to see the film. I had heard a lot about it, about the fact that it had been cut a lot due to its violence and touchy subject matter. I didn't like violent films as a rule, but this wasn't 'yobbish' violence or gangster culture, this was about a couple of twisted mass murderers on a joy ride across America. This was, and turned out to be, a great movie. It said a lot about how, in the media, serial killers become personalities. Kill a few people in a bizarre and motiveless fashion and you will be known and spoken about for years. Fame is at your fingertips. One line to cross and you will be there... crossing lines. Life is cheap...

I put my hand on Erica's leg and she did not make any attempt to move it. It wasn't quite holding hands but it fooled me into thinking this was not just a meeting, this was a date. I guess, looking back on it, my own mind was to blame. She had always liked me and I just presumed that she still did. Just because we got on so well together didn't mean that we were going to be a couple, but here I was with my hand on her jeans. Here I was feeling this sexual chemistry with her, and it was all in my mind.

We left the cinema and we spoke about the film, we analysed it, we had both liked it, if 'like' is a word you can use for something that had been so affective. She invited me back to her house and I was keen to go. If this was the start of something I didn't want it to end yet, and I was enjoying being with her. I imagined kissing her and I wanted to do it. I walked close to her, we looked into each other's eyes and we smiled. I should have known better. For fuck sake why did I let my guard down?

Back at her house we drank coffee, sitting opposite each other over the kitchen table. We did not speak much, there were silences, something was wrong and then she dropped the bomb. She told me that she had a boyfriend.

My heart sank. I was devastated. It was like a kick in the teeth. It was like saying "Steve, you were right to keep away from girls, this is what they do." Damn I don't really know why it hit me so hard, it's not as though I were in love with her or anything. I guess it was just bad timing. I was very down and I was coming to a part of my life where it was kill or cure. I was at the crossroads and that night the sign was pointing to a future, things seemed to be heading in Erica's direction and I had begun to walk down that road. I was planning a future for myself and when I got there I was told 'don't bother'. I had nowhere else to go. It was the one little knock I needed to send me over the edge.

We parted with very few words. She knew that I had been hurt by it, but she hadn't really done anything to lead me on, it had all been in my mind. My mind, as always, was my worst enemy.

As I walked the dark streets back towards the train station my mind darkened to a point I had never known before. I knew my mind well, I knew that it could become dark, but this was something new. I was talking to myself through clenched teeth, words I don't remember now, words that were forcing my decisions. I went into an off license and bought four cans of cider like a zombie doing something it remembered from an old life. I was on autopilot but the program was going wrong.

Somehow I made it home but it wasn't quick enough for me. I wanted to be in my room yet I had to travel on trains and on foot. My house was in the distance yet seemed to be getting further and further from my body. The bag of ciders was getting heavy and I could hardly wait to get the first one to my lips. Let me get home, and then it would start, then it would end.

I let myself into the house and could not avoid the unwelcome presence of my mother and her boyfriend. She came out of the lounge and stopped me from making my get away up the stairs. She asked me how the night went and I said, "ok" through gritted teeth. Her boyfriend was hovering in the background, a strange over intrusive character that had been on the scene for over a year. I could never judge what he was thinking or what he might do next. I begged that he would not speak to me; I longed to be away from them both. After a minute of discomfort I made it up to my bedroom and shut the door.

I used the dimmer switch that I had managed to convince my mother to put in my room, giving me just a dull light, which I preferred. You can't see what I look like in that light, nothing bright can get in. I opened a cider and took a long sip of the crisp cold liquid. I always liked cider because it tasted so alcoholic that you knew it would soon get you drunk. Beer was not as spiky. I fell into sitting on the floor with my knees pulled up to my chest and there I sat and thought and drunk. I think I knew what I was going to do but I didn't quite know what order to do things in. I wanted to get drunk, but there was something even more important than that. I wanted to die.

Was it all the love affairs that were going on around me that made my mind so sick? …Winona leaving me for another guy, my sister happy with her man, my mother happy with hers, Mickey and Mallory driving across America with a couple of rifles and matching wedding rings. Was it that I really didn't think much of life and was told on that very night that my feelings were correct? …That movie that showed how expendable life was, that girl showing me how wrong I was to think that life could be better. I was just this; useless, unwanted. …A mirage of a person. I can't quite put my finger on why it happened that night, but it happened all the same. Soon enough I was heading downstairs to the bathroom medicine cabinet and taking the box of co-proxomal tablets back to my room.

I bolted the door.

There was no question as to whether I would do this or not, it was unchangeable, it was set, it was my destiny.

I thought about watching 'Bram Stoker's Dracula' one more time before I died. I even put the video on and started watching it before I realised how redundant it was. It did not matter to me that these were my final hours. I wanted it done, I wanted to go. There was nothing that I thought of to keep me from that final decision. I was not going to miss anything. I had not got anything in my life that was worth living for. This was total, my thoughts focused. I was going to die.

I listened to Annie Lennox singing the song 'No More I Love Yous'. That song seemed to fit my mood and I had bought the single recently despite the fact that it did not really fit into the music category I would usually listen to or would be expected to listen to. I must have played it twenty times before the night was done. I played it over and over. I cracked open the pills and let them fall into a pile on my black bed sheets. I drank more cider as I sat on my bedroom floor and stared at the pills. I didn't wait long. I hadn't got a decision to make; it was already too late for me. I put four or five of the pills into my mouth and swallowed them down with the cider. Then, without any further thought I did it again and again until the pills were all gone. They were all in my body. They would now go about their business of killing me, but I had taken about fifty and nothing was happening.

I sat there for a while waiting for death to come to me but I grew impatient. My mother and her boyfriend had gone to bed, completely unaware of what I was doing. I went downstairs again to see if there was anything else I could take. I found a few travel sickness pills and I took them. Then I took a swig of cough syrup before staggering back to my room and the darkness within.

I wrote a note, a page long note about how bad my life was, about how I could not cope with emotions and rejections and the perpetual feeling of dark despair. I truly thought that it would be the last thing I ever wrote. It seemed so important to say exactly how I felt so that my family would understand. I wanted them to forgive me and wanted them to see that there was no other solution for me, that I really had no choice. The note has been lost completely and that is probably for the best. I know that when you are in the 'suicide zone' you do not speak or write anything rational. What I wrote that night was probably pathetic and embarrassing, if I read it now I would probably cringe.

I lay on the bed now; I crossed my arms like a corpse in its coffin and waited. I waited there staring at my room, at the posters of bands I once liked to listen to and movies I once liked to watch. None of it mattered anymore. Nothing changed my mind. At no stage did I regret what I had done or think that I might actually survive, but survive I did.

I awoke to screams through my bedroom door. "What have you done...? Steve answer me...", but my mother obviously knew exactly what I had done. She had obviously gone to her medicine cabinet and found the box of painkillers missing. Perhaps this was not as much of a shock to her as it was to me. Perhaps she had been waiting for this day.

I got up and nearly fell back down again. My head swam like a tidal wave and my eyes blurred and darted around the room. I staggered and fell against my door, my palms on the black gloss paint, my eyes searching. I could see the glistening silver bolt; my head dizzier than any alcohol could ever induce. My eyes span despite my instructions to concentrate on that lock. The voice of my mother's cries rang in my ears and I couldn't answer, my tongue twisted in my mouth, my words slurred to the point of incomprehension. I grabbed the bolt and I twisted it but only managed to screw off one part of it, leaving the door bolted shut. I tried to tell my mother that I couldn't do it but I couldn't form a word, and then I did it and the door swung open. I fell into my mother's arms and she held me up, keeping me walking while her boyfriend phoned for an ambulance.

I was in a daze and I can hardly remember what happened next, the drugs still playing with my mind. I know I was taken into the ambulance and they were asking what I had taken, then we were moving and I lay back on the stretcher. At the hospital I was sick and things were stuck in my arms. People were talking to me and I think I gave them an answer in some slurred response. Nurses were all around me and I lay there as they came and went. I worried that some of my old work colleges would see me. I remember waiting a long time for anything to happen. I was still wearing the clothes I had worn the night before and felt very overdressed to be lying in hospital. I guess I hadn't planned this part.

The next thing I remember is waking up in the ward attached to drips and with my mother and her boyfriend sitting at my side. They tried to be caring but there is only so much compassion you can have for something so self inflicted. My mother wanted to know one thing only and she said it again and again... 'Why?'

It was a question that I couldn't really answer. I could have blamed the whole thing on Erica but if it weren't her it would have only been someone or something else. I had been waiting for an excuse and when it came I took it with open arms. ...But all I knew now was that I had done it and that it had not worked. What did it take to get out of this? What was I supposed to feel now? Well, my mother knew something that I didn't and that I would never be told. Apparently they had told her that I could still die, that my liver could have been irreparably damaged. I could go at any moment and so I lay there staring at the demons that circled around the curtains like so many self induced acid trips, blissfully unaware of the damage I had caused. ...Damage to my own life and damage to the lives of my family.

The curtains were patterned with orange spirals and each one of them became a grimacing face staring back at me. My body felt like a thousand little pins were digging into my flesh, tingling and sending shooting pains to the ends of every nerve. My head felt like it was in a bubble and I couldn't shake it free. I felt broken.

People were talking to me. My mother's boyfriend was saying something like a buzzing insect in my ear. My mother looked as broken as I was. My sister came and looked so confused and hurt. I just lay there wishing the bed would suck me down and take me away from them all.

I think that surviving a suicide attempt is the worst feeling ever. You had felt bad enough to make that decision, you had managed to pluck up the courage to do something about it, yet here you still are feeling equally if not more depressed than you were before. You wish so much that it had just worked so that you did not have to live through this yet you feel so ill that the idea of trying again is abhorrent. You feel completely trapped in your own body and there appears to be no way out. Yet you have been given another chance. Your soul was not accepted into heaven or hell or where ever it was trying to get to and here you are, trying to see a way to go on from this.

I think I managed to see it as positive. I decided that I would not try it again but that I would accept it as something to learn from, something to make me stronger. Even though the blood tests had come back and I was given the all clear, I was not allowed to leave. I had to talk with psychiatrists so that they could assess if I was still a risk and whether I was a complete loony or not. Half of me wanted to be declared as insane so that I could be locked away in hospital and not have to work or function in the real world ever again. But part of me wanted some kind of a life back, a life much changed from the one I had been living.

"I believe you quite seriously wanted to die didn't you?"

"Yes."

"What happened to make you feel this way?"

"Nothing." What did they want? A bloody list?

"What happened that night that was different to any other night?"

I didn't want Erica to get the blame. I didn't want to give her the satisfaction of being the only cause when there was so much more involved than that. I didn't want to mention my skin lest they just think I was terribly vain. I was embarrassed by my reasons, yet I knew that there were deeper ones. I had been depressed for years and something just had to give. So I just told them I had felt down, that I just didn't want to be alive.

"Do you see any reason to live?"

"No."

"Are you planning to try again?"

"No."

...And so they allowed me to go - spat back out into the same old world that I had tried to escape from which now looked so new to me. It wasn't quite as stale and unwelcome as it had been before. I had crawled back out of the pit, over the peak, and now I could live again. I would go to therapy and I would take the drugs that they had prescribed for me and perhaps that was enough to make things better. Perhaps drugs and chatting to mental health professionals was all I needed. I had been given Prozac and I had been allocated a therapist but really that was all they could do. They could not change my life, they could not make me want to live, I would have to do that myself. Perhaps I could make it change. Perhaps I could have a life.

I remember walking around Hitchin town and looking at all the people thinking, "they don't know that I am the walking dead - that I have come back from the brink". I felt more alive than I had felt in years. I wasn't happy, but I knew that I could be. I didn't want to be dead, yet I didn't want that same old life. I needed things to change, and I hoped and believed that they would. I was in control. I would have to start making some changes.

Pretty soon after that I had my first tattoo and, I thought at the time, the only tattoo I wanted. It was a bat with a bleeding heart in the centre. It seemed to sum up the way I was feeling as well as my personality and love for vampires. It was a statement about what had happened to me, a physical scar for a mental wound. Now, thirteen years on. I am covered in tattoos.

<u>Self Harming</u>

I wanted everything to be different but it just wasn't. My life had been turned upside down yet no one could see it. My family was acting as if nothing had happened. I didn't tell my friends. Part of me wanted to yell it from the rooftops but it just isn't done, to tell people. People wouldn't know how to deal with such information; no one knows what to say. I guess that's why we have therapists. I was on a waiting list to see someone with the Hitchin mental health department, a wait that would take over a month. In that time I could have gone flying off the rails again. If a therapist was there to save me, then shouldn't they see me as soon as possible? Someone that has failed a suicide attempt must surely be at the top of the endangered list? I guess not.

I went straight back to the life I had been having before, unemployed, obsessed with my appearance, nothing to occupy my mind but my own despair. I was still counting calories, feeling guilty for every slice of bread that passed my lips afraid that I would grow fat. Still I had to spend time in front of the mirror each morning just so that I could face myself, despite the fact that no one but my mother was likely to see me. I was still fanatical about weight training each night. It felt like my body and face were out of my control and I was constantly fighting to get that control back. If I ate too much, I would weight train for longer. If I missed a night of training, I would starve myself the next day, but I tried to keep to routine and that's all my life was.

My social life did still exist. I still went out to see bands at the local venues spending literally hours in front of the mirror applying my make up and styling my hair so that I could be seen. I still wished that I would meet someone to fill the void. There were still fleeting moments where things seemed ok, but they hardly cancelled out my perpetual low moods. There were times when I thought I might have met a girl and times when they seemed to be laughing in my face. I really didn't think I had a chance with anyone - I was too crazy - too hung up about everything. If I were to meet someone they would soon find out what I was really like and dump me on the spot.

That wasn't just theory - that was fact. It happened and it set me right back. I was making lunch in the kitchen when the phone rang. It was the girl I had seen a few times, a relationship that never seemed to get off the ground, but I had told her too much. I had let her know some of my fears, some of my life, and she couldn't deal with it. She wanted sex and I couldn't deliver. She had rung me to say that she didn't want to see me again. I shouldn't have been overly bothered but having an excuse to take another overdose was just too much of a temptation. My suicidal urge was always there just waiting for the right buttons to be pressed; laying dormant ready for an eruption. I left the lunch half made on the kitchen sideboard and went to the bathroom to get the pills.

There was a box of co-proxamol tablets in the medicine cabinet just as there always was. Didn't my mother care that I might do it again? Why hadn't she hidden all the medication away from me? Surely that would have been the sensible thing to do? Surely you should not leave strong painkillers in the reach of a depressed teenager who had once nearly killed themselves with them? Perhaps my mother didn't care as much as she made out. Or perhaps she, along with everyone else, just didn't understand this at all.

The box had about fifty tablets in it but I just took a few strips out. I didn't want my mother to notice that they had gone missing, but if I was planning to die why did it matter if my mother noticed a few tablets missing out of the cupboard? Well in hindsight I can only imagine that this latest bout of suicidal behaviour was just a cry for help. I hadn't exactly had much help had I? Was it too much to ask that someone do something for me since I nearly died?

I think I took about twenty tablets. It felt like another suicide attempt yet if I had reasoned it all out, I would have known that it wouldn't work. I hadn't taken nearly enough, yet I went upstairs and lay on my bed and waited for death all the same. How dare that girl not want to be with me? It wasn't my fault that I was depressed, but being depressed had really begun to make me miserable. Let it all end. Please God... Surely, if you exist at all, surely you must see that I am really serious about this whole death thing. I had tried it once so now I was trying it again. Just take me for Christ' sake!

I think I slept for a while but I was soon awake and feeling very ill. It was like coming down off acid and alcohol together...a hang over with delirium. I staggered downstairs and tidied up the kitchen ready for my mother's return from work priding myself on my foresight that had told me not to take too many of her pills. Hopefully she would not notice a thing.

When she came home from work I pretended that everything was fine. She made a dinner of bacon and eggs and I sat there eating it with my stomach churning. I took a mouthful before the end, and I rushed off my chair and threw it all up in the toilet. I said that I was feeling unwell and I went up to bed. I never told her. That little attempt at my life just became another dark secret for me to harbour. I don't think I told anybody. If it was a cry for help it hadn't worked.

The next day I felt as though my stomach had been scraped and my head was fuzzy. I decided that I should go to the doctor's just in case I had done myself some serious damage. I went in and up to the desk. The place was heaving with sick people and I felt very much on show. I wanted them all to disappear. I wanted to be the only one there, just me and the doctor...sterile. I couldn't deal with these feelings of depression, social phobia and illness all at once. I thought that I might go mad and thought of running out.

The lady at the desk said that she was 'very sorry' but they were fully booked and I would have to come back tomorrow. I couldn't believe it. I sought help and again it was denied. Was there no one that was going to help me through this? I felt like yelling out and bashing my head against the wall. "Can't you see I need help? I might die! I took a fucking overdose!", but no one wanted to hear it. No one wanted to help.

I never did go back to the doctor's because the next day I felt much better physically. I was far from well though. Mentally I was a long cry from ok and I had to find a way to deal with it.

I somehow came to the conclusion that I should cut my skin. There had been times that I had cut myself with a pair of compasses at school but I never thought much about it. I did it because I was bored. I cut a pentagram into my wrist because I was interested in Satan and thought it was cool. I surely hope that Satan doesn't exist because I sold my soul to him a few times while I was at school, but this was different. I was angry with myself for being so useless. I hated myself. I hated the way I looked and I hated my life. I took a pair of scissors and I held them tight in my right hand with the blades closed and facing down. Then I did it. Savagely and quickly I slashed the back of my left wrist; all my anger, all my hate, all that self-loathing lashing out. The pain was sharp and refreshing. Still my mind felt set to burst, full as it was of so much hatred. I sat and stared at the grazes I had made and was pleased to see little beads of blood oozing out from each red scratch. Then I did it again and again until the anger had subsided, and then I just sat there on the bathroom floor and watched the blood come. I sat there for ages getting my breath back and staring at the wounds I had made. I sat there until my mind calmed down and then I licked all the blood off my arm and left the bathroom.

This was different to carving stars in your arm to impress your friends. I was cutting myself now because it was the only way I could deal with my feelings. This was a need and after I had done it the urge to do it had subsided and I felt quite contented to have done this for myself. However, now I would have to wear long sleeves to cover the scars and the blood. I had to keep this secret. I didn't know that this was a symptom of depression and no one had ever really diagnosed me as depressed anyway. I was going through my illness blind and flailing.

Eventually I did get to speak with a therapist and we sat there going over my childhood and school days and anything else that I thought might be important. The therapist was a lady far into her middle ages who sat quite still with a clipboard on her lap tapping a biro against the page. I spoke about my feelings and about my life. I told her things I had never told anyone and I was waiting for her reaction, waiting for her to put it all into perspective for me and tell me what one thing during my upbringing had sparked all this off. But she said nothing. Occasionally she would write something down but then just look back up at me urging me to continue. She asked me questions; I answered them. I told her about my writing and about the things I did enjoy despite the apathy I felt about most of my life. I told her all the things that I believed could have made me this way but at no point did she say, "Yes, that's it, that's why." She didn't really do anything at all - I did it. I was speaking myself into submission.

Maybe getting all those things out of my mind and into open air helped disperse them a little. Maybe the therapist did her job perfectly. After a few months I was ready to go it alone, as long as I kept taking the Prozac; I was given the all clear. She said that I was a young, intelligent young man with a lot to live for and, quite honestly, I believed her. I guess the pills were working. I had left the edge of my dark pit and although I could still see it I was not going to fall. I stopped seeing the therapist after just a few visits.

The next big thing to happen came only about a month later. I was twenty now, an age that I hated, as it seemed to mean that I was no longer a teenager and had to become a responsible adult. I think I felt that my age was overtaking my maturity and while I spent all my time depressed my life was slipping away. My twentieth birthday sucked and I can't remember enjoying any birthday since.

Summer had come and the Hitchin 'Triangle festival' was a place to sit on the grass, drink alcohol and listen to live music. I met Rick there and he was with a bunch of people, some of which I had met, some I hadn't. There was a girl there that seemed to know a few of Rick's friends but she would come and go between talking to them and then going away with her own friend. I guess I was interested in her but I was not focusing on any one thing that day. I felt good. I liked the warmth of the sun. I liked the 20/20 red wine that I was sipping from the bottle. I looked my best and felt free. I remember that my sister and her boyfriend were there. They had been together some years and had a child, my little niece who I adored. I remember running around with her on my shoulders and flitting between my family and my friends. The alcohol was making me lose my inhibitions. I didn't remember to feel depressed or to act any certain way. I was myself, the best I ever was, and I didn't wish to be any different.

The girl I had been interested in came back to our little group and I managed to include her in the conversation. She seemed quite feisty; a polite way to say that she had a superiority complex and didn't seem to be concerned with trying to impress anyone. She had impressed me. I found out that her name was Carey and I hoped that I could get to speak to her properly at some stage but she didn't really show any interest in me. She didn't seem interested in anyone, but I was focused now, the effects of the alcohol making anything seem possible, even the chance of Stephen Westwood meeting a nice girl.

When the evening came the crowd at the festival thinned out a little and we found out that there was an alternative disco/club night at the local venue just five minutes walk from the field. We decided to go there. As we walked down the darkening street so did a lot of others that obviously had the same idea. One of those others was Carey. I decided to act on it.

I quickened my pace and caught up with her and there we were, walking together and chatting about the day and about music and about God knows what. I was drunk but I was in perfect control. Yet I was doing something that I never did, I was chatting up a girl, and it seemed to be working. I was being myself but I didn't tell her anything that might put her off me. My white silk shirt was covering the fresh cuts on my wrist. I kept the conversation light and glossed around any talk about me. I found out all I could about her.

She had only just finished school and was sixteen, but I felt quite immature for a twenty year old so that didn't seem like such a big gap. I had not had much experience with girls and my naivety kept my dating age right down. What did I have to offer someone of my own age? I had no job, I couldn't drive, and I didn't know what I was doing sexually. It was just as well she was young, young girls might still fall for the facade of 'coolness' that I, arguably, portrayed.

She was very petite and her hair was light brown with dashes of blond that waved slightly and finished just above her shoulders. Her face was small, her nose short

74

and her lips thin. Her skin was fresh with a few freckles. She wore a long skirt with Dr. Marten boots and a Rage Against The Machine T-Shirt. I was attracted to her, she had the look I liked, alternative but not for the sake of being so. She seemed to be her own person.

I liked her and her relative lack of interest in me made me like her more. I couldn't tell - did she like me at all? Well she was talking to me. I was making her smile and even making her laugh. I don't remember what we had to talk about. The thought of having to attempt to chat someone up now fills me with dread, and I know it did then as well; it must have been the wine that softened my neuroses. I was chatting to her all the way to the club and then, as we piled through the one small door I lost her.

More drink and laughs with Rick and his friends must have relaxed me a lot because there was one rule that I had when going to clubs and that was that on no account did I dance. Well, Carey appeared and she held out her hand asking me to get up and dance with her and I did it. I got up, went out onto the crowded dance floor and began to move to the music. I kept the moving down to a minimum lest I make a complete fool of myself in front of someone I was trying to impress, but I did it and did it for quite some time. She danced well I thought, letting herself go and skipping on the spot. I did some old fashioned Goth thing with my hands. I obviously hadn't frightened her off with my incompetence because when I asked for her number at the end of the night she gave it to me quite happily and even allowed me to walk her and her friend to the train station.

That was the end of what I thought to myself was a very successful day and I caught a taxi and made my way home quite pleased with myself.

The next day was Sunday and I paced around the house fighting with my emotions. I was excited to have met someone but I still had that basic self preservation that told me all girls were a bad idea and I would only end up getting hurt. I should have listened to my instincts. Telling my mother was not the best thing I could have done. She was urging me to make the call and saying how bad it would be of me to not call her after I said that I would. That was playing on my conscience. I wasn't the kind of guy that meets a girl and then stands her up or just doesn't get in touch at all. I was the kind of guy that was searching for love and just wanted to have a girlfriend. Or was I? Was I not a depressed guy that should be concentrating on his own problems and not making extra ones? Had I not, only a few months before, attempted to kill myself? Could I actually be in a fit state to tackle the emotional world of dating?

After a whole day of uncertainty and battles in my head; after a whole day of plucking up the courage to speak with this relative stranger completely sober, I called the number. Her mother answered and I asked to speak with Carey. It wasn't a fake number. Her voice said 'hello' quite confidently down the line. It was a little awkward, but not overly, and we spoke for long enough to prove that we were both still interested and made a date to meet at Bowes Lion where some bands were playing that coming Friday. It was done. I had a date.

The night of the date went really well. I had spent the usual two hours getting ready but I had not overly panicked and, once we were together, it was that we were going to be girl and boyfriend. We liked similar things and spent a lot of the time watching and analysing other people picking apart their characters and their looks. I did that so much in my head that talking about others in that way was really good fun no matter how mean it truly was. It felt that I had met someone on a similar wavelength to myself; someone that didn't go through life blindly. She liked Nirvana and some other bands that, although not favourites of mine, still held credibility. It still showed that she thought about emotions and didn't just go through her life blindly. I felt that we might be kindred spirits.

What else did I like about her? It is hard to remember now with such years of bitterness between now and then. I don't even want to think about all that was good between us because it was all a lie. Of course, I felt much differently at the time. I was taken in by her. I hadn't got a picture of the sort of girl I wanted to meet but I was sure that she was it. She attached our hands together with the links off a beer four pack and I didn't try to escape.

We were happily going through the excitement that comes with getting to know a new person of the opposite sex. I no longer rode my scooter after having a bad accident on it that had broken my wrist and broken my bike. I didn't really trust it again. I used to ride a mountain bike to go and see Carey - riding all the way from Wymondley to Stevenage and staying in her room until her mother called us, saying "it's getting late", which meant I had to go. Her parents didn't mind us being alone together but we had only played around sexually. I still had my doubts about the whole thing. I doubted whether I could do it and doubted that I wanted to. Sex was bound to rear its ugly head at some stage and I was waiting for that time with dread and wonder.

Carey seemed to suffer with a mild depression that could easily have just been teenage angst. After a while I did tell her that only months before I had attempted suicide and instead of running a mile or showing any shock she told me about her own feelings. It felt easier to have told her; it was one less dark secret to carry on my shoulders; but there were other skeletons in my closet and if we continued to get close they would start to come screaming out.

Carey told me how she had cut a few times and we talked about it at length. It seems it isn't so unusual. Cutting is just a way to cope with unwanted emotion. It is like having a good cry, getting a fluid out of your body that somehow seems to carry your feelings. Afterwards you feel relieved like you have managed to outrun your emotion although you know it's still on your tail.

Carey said that she wanted to get away from everything, how she wanted to run away from her parents and her life, and I, with a more mature head, suggested that we go on holiday. She jumped at the chance and we started to look through camping brochures for somewhere to go. Her parents, she said, would drive us to the site if it was not too far away and I knew that we could use my sister's tent. It seemed like a romantic idea. It seemed that we would get a break from life, but Carey said once we had decided where to go, "I'm not going to sleep with you."

I was taken back by the directness but was not overly disappointed or annoyed or anything negative, just surprised. I had been thinking that if we went together like that it was bound to happen whether I wanted it to or not. Well she told me that it would not happen and I accepted that. I was in no rush - I wasn't that kind of guy. I was scared of that happening and ruining what we had. Little did I know that I would be afraid like that for years.

Carey was a virgin and so was I. I understood if she felt awkward about it because I felt like that too. I, no doubt, felt worse than most and it didn't happen. We went on this camping trip to the country; to a place I can't even remember now, with no money and with just the bare minimum of food. We just wanted to be there away from everyone and everything else. We spent a lot of time talking. We played a few games of Battleships. We listened to music on a little battery-operated stereo. We went for walks in the fields full of cows and shit. We lived together. We kissed in the way you do when you have only been together a while, just wanting our lips to be together. We went through our life stories. We were two kids on the brink of love. We didn't have any idea what the future held, but it seemed that things were good. She was lulling me into a state of security that I would be fooled by for years.

So I had a girlfriend. I had someone to talk to, someone to hold me, someone to share things with. I was told by another human being that I was loved - LOVED! She said it in French first as I left one night on my bike. We kissed good-bye and she said it and I biked away, not entirely sure what she had just said yet pretty much convinced that it must have been love. I pedaled home excited and happy. My depression was nearly gone and I was thankful for the Prozac. It seemed that the drugs were taking the edge off my despair and this girl was holding my hand, leading me to a better future.

Is love all we need? Is love all I need? It certainly helps. Here was someone telling me that I was good enough to be with. I was being told that I was funny, that I was sweet, that I was kind, that I was cool. I was being shown that I was good looking enough to want to kiss. Yet I was being told that I was not good enough to make love to. It just went on like that. She made me feel bad for even thinking that something was wrong. "Is that what defines love for you?" she would ask me once and I couldn't answer. I wasn't dying to lose my virginity; I was still afraid of it, but I knew that it was just something that two people in love did - they made love. Well Carey and I did not.

At first we would go out together to the places I used to go to. We went to Bowes Lion to see bands just as I always had. Carey had friends, I had friends and we would all hang out together. Sometimes we would just go to a playground and drink alcohol and have a laugh. I started the band back up and we did gigs every so often and Carey would be cheering from the crowd. She wanted to be with someone that was a drummer in a punk band. She wanted to be on the arm of this older, alternative looking guy. At least I thought that she did.

I was quite in touch with myself at that age. I knew what I had been through, and what I had been. I was twenty. I was fully grown in body and mind. I wasn't still trying to find myself, I had found him, and here I was. I was a Goth. I dressed in black and dyed my hair. I listened to the Cure and the misfits. I was 'Vampire Steve' and that was who Carey liked wasn't it? That was whom she loved. Well, time would prove otherwise.

The only thing that seemed to be wrong at first was that I was lacking money. I had spent most of my childhood savings account on going out and on alcohol. I had to get a job and Carey was urging me to do so. That was the next stage of my life and I knew it had to be done. I scoured the newspaper looking for something that I might be able to do with my complete lack of skills. Something I could do despite my disaster at the hospital. Eventually I came across an advert for a warehouse operative in Letchworth and it didn't say that I needed any particular skills. My sights were not set high, I had no ambition, and it seemed just fine. So I went for it.

I put my hair in a ponytail, slicked down the top that I usually back combed into a bird's nest, wore a shirt and trousers and went for an interview. I got the job. I was filled with equal portions of hope and despair. Here I was being given a chance, and here I was beginning a life of mediocrity.

It wasn't bad at first. I was good at the job and, like a subject at school, when you are good at something you like it more. I was just picking orders but I did it well and, although I knew the people there thought I was weird, I got on ok with the other staff members.

My relationship with Carey was going fine until one winter's night that we, along with Rick, went to a club in Hitchin where they had an alternative disco. I had been

80

dropped off by my mother and met both of them at the train station. They seemed very friendly with each other and it seemed that we might have a good night. I had dressed up, they had dressed down, but that was just our way. I always took hours to get ready where as Rick for instance would just wear a T-shirt and jeans. I know he hated the way he looked but it didn't stop him from enjoying himself. He was thin with long blond hair and he had quite bad skin. I never saw that when I looked at him - to me he was just Rick - a good friend and the bass player in my band, but I know he always felt inferior to me in the looks department. If only he had known how dreadful my phobias were. If only he knew how insecure I was about my own appearance. Little did he know that he had it much better than me.

We walked together to the club, which was not far, and started an evening of drinking and chatting on the leather sofa they had in the corner, but something was not right. The chatting seemed to mainly be between Carey and Rick, I just sat there with little to say, hating the place for all its loud music, people trying to get off and get drunk. So I decided the only way I would be able to enjoy all this was if I were to drink and lose my sober phobias. I got a snake bite and proceeded to drink pint after pint of the stuff, stewing in my own juices. I hated the people, I hated the noise. I was getting too old for this shit; I guess I was thinking that I was too old for Carey. I guess she would be better off with someone that can enjoy themselves at these places and there she was, chatting and laughing with Rick. Let them get on with it - I'd had enough.

Carey was talking to some guy by the pool table and I just saw red. I saw everything me and Carey had just thrown out the window. I stormed out of the club and Carey came running after me. I said that I just needed to be alone, I raced away without letting her talk, I got into a taxi and I went home.

It wasn't until I was home that I realised I had Carey's stuff in my pockets. I had her make up and I had her purse. I would have to see her again to give her those things back but at the moment I didn't want her at all. Perhaps I had over reacted. Perhaps I was just insecure and felt bad because she was not giving me enough reassurance. Or perhaps she had got bored of me and wanted Rick.

She phoned me the next day with poison on her tongue. She shouted down the phone at me, telling me that Rick had got no money and that they had been stranded in Hitchin all night. It was below freezing and they had tried to sleep under a bush on Windmill Hill. All I could think of was them two hugging each other to keep warm. Yes I felt guilty for causing them so much discomfort but part of me knew that they deserved it for the way they had treated me. Perhaps they had sex. Perhaps Rick was good enough to sleep with. Perhaps I should just leave them to it.

We split up over that. Carey told me that she did not think we should continue seeing each other. Perhaps she wanted to be seeing Rick, I didn't know. I was back to being alone yet I felt more alone than ever. We should have been together yet there I was, back in my room, back to drinking cider alone and listening to Radiohead, an album I had copied from Carey. Those songs still remind me of that split from her. Words to those songs became the soundtrack to my depression. 'You do it to yourself, that's what really hurts'. I was cutting myself in my mother's bathroom with a Stanley blade stolen from work. I drew a heart and a 'C' on my inner wrist. One night I took the blade out in my room and concentrated hard as I carved the words 'end the pain' across the back of my wrist. I wanted her to know. I wanted her to see the pain she had caused me. The mental pain now a physical one as the blood seeped out of my wounds. It hurt at first but after a while it felt sweet, deserved, like a tattoo. I lay down and stared at the wound, watching the blood dry. I curled up in a ball on my bed safe in my dark pit once again.

Trouble was, I had all this pain yet I had a job to hold down. I still had to go in every day after a night of bleeding and drinking and restless sleep. I had to wear long sleeves so that they could not see my cuts and when I went to lift a box off a high shelf, my sleeve would fall down and 'End the pain' would be visible in scabs on my skin. No one said anything. One night at home I 'scribbled' over the words in my arm with a blade. I erased it into a mess across my skin so that it could not be seen as words anymore. I bled and felt that she had done this to me, that it was all Carey's fault.

Days and weeks went by with this weighing me down. All day I did the job thinking of suicide. Every train that I heard go past was another reminder that I wanted to be in front of it, stubbing out my pain. I planned another overdose. I planned to slit my wrists, yet I was going to work each day and pretending things were normal. My mind was everywhere but on the job. I was constantly thinking about how I could make things right with Carey. I was thinking that if I couldn't then there was always the trains. Every night I would get a bottle of Turbo white cider and drink myself to sleep.

It was around this time that I chose another tattoo. I decided that I wanted a fallen angel and after a little time of searching for an appropriate picture I remembered that there was a good angel picture on one of my albums. I had the album on vinyl, the picture showing an angel kissing a devil while stabbing him in the back. It said it all, and once I had decided to get it done it felt like a burning need. I felt naked without it, I felt stupid that I only had one small tattoo and felt that my body just didn't say enough about me. So I had it done, three sessions of pain and a work of art was on my skin. I was very proud of it and showed it off to everyone at work. I wanted to tell Carey about it. I wondered if she would like it.

Things got a little obsessive. I would bike to Carey's house and sit under a tree staring at her bedroom window. I would see the light on in there and I would think about her and of what we once had. I looked up there imagining what she might be doing, wondering if she thought of me at all. I sat there and then, when her light went off, I would bike back home.

Eventually I plucked up courage to knock on her door and she allowed me in to speak with her. For three hours I sat on her stairs with her and told her how much I loved her. I said that we should be together and that I was sorry for jumping to conclusions, that I was just depressed and everything was magnified for me. None of it was lies. My emotional state was so fragile that I could not cope with anything. I could not cope if Carey and I were apart. I begged her to reconsider.

It seemed to be working. She said that she still loved me and there seemed to be no reason to remain separated from each other. We swore from then on to be with each other and to talk about everything and not allow anything to split us up. It was only later that I found out that she had actually been out with Rick and another guy while we were separated. It was only I that had been locked in his room with his cider and his music. She had been living her teenage life, dating people on the rebound; dating my best friend.

My mother could see how depressed I was and she didn't think that Carey was helping. Yet I did not listen to her, I guess you just don't listen to your mother when you are that age even though you may still live with her. I was too old for mothering yet not old enough to be wise. We were at each other's throats all the time. I spent all my time in my room and barely communicated with her anymore. Living in the same house as my mother was getting me down. I wanted to have my own life yet there were still these rules and these opinions being thrown at me. Carey was the same, although younger than me, she had reached that age where she hated her parents and wanted to be free of them...The answer? We decided to move in together.

It could be argued that this was not such a good idea. It could be said that only a few weeks before we had split up over my stupid jealousy. It could be said that on the miserly wage I was earning we would not be able to have a good house or a good life. It could be said that we had no furniture or money to get any. It could have been said that I was not well enough to deal with the adult world. Lots of things could be and were said, but two young adults in love have there own views, which are a damn sight stronger than common sense. The more we were told that we could not do it the more we decided that we would.

We managed to secure a flat that would be paid for by housing benefit and all bills would be paid for out of my wages. We would be poor but we would be together. How romantic that sounded, but how dull it really was. I was constantly unhappy. I worked ridiculously long hours at work to get the over time money. I would leave at seven in the morning to get a lift with a work colleague and the work would go on until it was finished, nine, ten sometimes as late as midnight. I was tired and depressed. I remember nights lying on the bed (we had no sofa) just saying, "we will never get out of this, we will never have any money". We ate toast and pasta for dinner and never went out. It was hardly living the dream, but nothing was going to stop us being together. It didn't matter that our relationship was more like that of a brother and a sister. We hardly even kissed anymore. We hugged in bed but it seemed so innocent. There was never any chance of sexual contact. She was my younger sibling and I looked after her as best I could. The thing was that no one was looking after me. I was still ill, despite massive improvements, I wasn't having any fun and though it wasn't nearly as bad as before, I still worried about my face. I had stolen some make up from the shop, too embarrassed to go up to the counter with it, and I tried to keep it secret from Carey. I had to do my make up every morning before Carey could see me and I did it before bed at night, sometimes spending ages in the bathroom picking at my skin hoping that I could turn the bedroom light off before I entered the room. Life was much harder than it needed to be, and it was glaringly obvious that Carey and I should not have been together.

What do you do to make a sour relationship more exciting? You have a child. Well Carey had come to the conclusion that we should have a kid. I don't know what my own views were on the subject. During those years I don't know what my views were about anything as they were always swallowed up by Carey's. I did what I thought would please her. I remember even thinking it to myself... "I live to make things nice for Carey. I live for her sake". I had no life. I was losing myself. The Stephen I had been was being diluted.

Well as far as I know there is only one way to have a child and that is to have sex. If we had a child it would be by Immaculate Conception and would make us a fortune. One night Carey and I lay together and she said that she wanted to make a baby and so we made the moves, we got undressed. Even that was something I was not used to. Carey always told me to look the other way when she got undressed and the sight of her naked body was not one I was used to, but I loved her. All this I put up with because I loved her. Didn't I? Or was I just looking after someone that so obviously needed my help.

There was no passion. We lay together but she did not touch me. The lights were out and I could only see her as a grey phantom lying on top of me. I tried to touch her sensually; I tried to do what I had seen on TV and read in

86

books. I tried to do what I thought she wanted and thought that I should do. I tried to make love to her, but we were both so awkward about it that there was no romance. There was no sexiness. I tried to do what I was supposed to but she said that it hurt and told me to stop. It was a total disaster and she just got off me and said that she didn't want to anymore and I was left in the room alone, rejected as always. I lay on the bed alone just wondering what was going through Carey's mind, convinced that she would blame me for being useless and that was as close as it got.

Why did we stay together through years of semi-love? Why did we see each other through such poverty and hard work? Carey became a photo processor and I continued to work hard at my job. We saw very little of each other and that was suiting me fine. I valued all the times that she was at work and I was not. Every Saturday I wrote, working on my first novel, dreading her coming home. Life with her was secular. She wasn't interested in having intellectual conversations. She thought that my writing was a waste of time. She told me off for using 'big words' that she did not understand. We were both getting older, becoming more attuned to who we were, yet I was being stifled by her and what she wanted. I wasn't changing. I was the same person I had always been yet somehow that just wasn't good enough for her anymore. She wanted me to be different and she let me know it all the time. I wanted to delve deeper into thoughts of the mind. She wanted to go to clubs and listen to God awful dance music. She dumped her former friends and wanted me to do the same. She made me quit the band again. She stopped me from seeing them. She told me to get off the Prozac and I did. She wanted me to dress differently - cut my hair and look fashionable and all I had to learn from was her. If she told me I looked awful in the clothes I was wearing then I believed her. If she told me that my hair would look better cut short then that's what I did. She was manipulating me and I was letting her because we were in love. Weren't we? I don't know if I even thought about such romantic ideas anymore. Romance was something that she did not give time to.

If this was my life, if she was growing up and growing away from what I had once loved, why then did this person become my wife? Was I so under the thumb that I thought there was nothing else in life worth striving for? Was I so dedicated to making someone else happy that I had forgotten about myself? Was my self-esteem so low that I didn't feel that I deserved more?

At her birthday I announced that there was one more present for her but that she could only have it on one condition. That present was a ring, an engagement ring, and when I showed her it and asked the inevitable question she said no. She did not want to marry me. Yet she wanted the ring - she loved the ring - and she took it and put it on her finger denying that it meant anything about marriage.

I didn't understand. I was not surprised or even that hurt, but I just didn't get it. Wasn't this what she wanted? Could I have been so wrong? What the hell was she doing with me anyway? I thought that she wanted someone to look after her. I thought that she wanted me.

Everything we once had in common was gone. Everything I loved about her had changed, as she had grown older. She had grown into who she was going to be and I still held on to the girl I had loved from the beginning. Fuck - she was still a child when I met her. The adult she had become had nothing in common with me. There was nothing between us worth saving. There was nothing between us at all. The fact that we had been together for five years only meant that we were both gluttons for punishment and starved of love. We were both afraid of loneliness, but that is no reason to be with someone. Of course there were things I loved about her - but if I was planning to spend all my time and all my years with someone, why did I choose someone that was so damaging?...So totally wrong? The only reason we were together was that we could not survive a break up. Having someone dependant on me was the only thing keeping me alive and so the reason I wanted to marry her was because I wanted to survive. I knew that if we split I would have nothing, and left with nothing I would probably kill myself. So, as an act of self-preservation, I married her.

We spoke about it after that day. We spoke about how we might do it and, blessed with new knowledge as to the possibilities, Carey said that she would marry me after all. She had only said no because she didn't want a normal wedding. She had only said no because she had not realised that you could get married abroad and that the whole thing could be like one amazing holiday. So she got into the whole idea and we started to make plans. We planned a three-week holiday to the Dominican Republic with a wedding in the second week. Her parents would come for the second week and my family would come for that week too and it would be great. It certainly sounded good.

Our families were pleased that we were getting married, they didn't question it. We had obviously been with each other long enough as far as they were concerned and so we had their blessings. If only they knew what a facade our relationship was, they would never have wanted us to take that big step, but Carey's mum and dad were quite happy. They liked me well enough as I had always been polite to them and proven myself to be able to look after their daughter. I don't really think they would have cared anyway - they both seemed to be emotionally dead and that's where Carey had learnt her ice maiden tendencies. My mother had never liked Carey because once I had met her I was at odds with her, but she and my Nan would come to the wedding anyway. The rest of my family either could not afford it or just didn't deem it important enough, but we did have the support of the families. It would be fine.

My father gave his blessing too. He had begun to take more of an interest in my life now that I was older. I don't think he really liked children but now I was an adult we could communicate. I don't think he ever really liked Carey either but he was happy if I was happy. I couldn't tell anyone the truth. I couldn't admit that I was not at all happy. I could not tell any of them about how badly I was being treated and I don't know if even I could see it at the time. Perhaps I thought it was how things were and that was that...Carey and I, in love, in hate, in whatever it was. It was us.

The wedding holiday was wonderful. The Dominican Republic is a gorgeous place with lush green jungles and a clear turquoise sea. I had only been abroad on holiday a couple of times before and nothing I had seen was anywhere near to the beauty of this. The very first night we were there we sat on the dark beach and watched a lightning storm light up the night's sky. There was no rain, the air was hot, yet there were the flashes and the bolts of electricity crashing to the ground. It was a humbling experience and would have been romantic had I been there with someone else. It seemed that romance was a fallacy, something they made up for the sake of songs. I may as well of been sitting alone on that beach. The beauty of it was a personal right of passage.

The holiday was all-inclusive and there were about ten different bars around the complex all serving cocktails and beer and there were two big restaurants for our meals. The whole place was right on the beach but there were also two swimming pools and a couple of Jacuzzis. It was an ideal place and we were looking forward to getting married there in a gazebo with a backdrop of the ocean. We were looking forward to dressing up and being watched by the other holiday makers. We were looking forward to drinking champagne and having our photos taken. Did we, I wonder, actually think about what would happen in our lives afterwards? Were we ever looking forward to actually being married? Man and wife.

By the time the family arrived we were already tanned and had already been on an excursion white water rafting. We could tell our family about the place, about where it was best to sit for drinking or eating. We could tell them of the crazy weather that was scolding hot all the time but sometimes broken by a tropical downpour. We could point out the lizards and the humming birds. We were already residents.

Then, came the wedding. I got ready in my room alone, styling my hair and putting on the clothes in total silence. I was calm and reposed. I wasn't excited, I wasn't scared. This was just something I was doing, part of my fate; this was what was supposed to happen. I had vowed to stick by Carey and I was marrying her. This was my life.

I wore black jeans, as I could not find any trousers that I liked, a white poet shirt and a dark red waistcoat. My hair had grown out and was now completely my own colour. This was another condition that Carey had put on me. She wanted to see my natural hair colour and wanted it natural for the wedding. So my hair was light brown and spiked up. I could have been anyone, but I was Stephen Westwood. I was Carey's interpretation of myself. I did not remove my three silver hoop earrings.

Since being with Carey and while on Prozac the issues I had about my face and body had softened considerably. I was terribly worried that my face would be spotty or red on the day of the wedding, but most days I would apply the make up sparingly and without panic. It never went away completely. I would still never leave the house without it on and every night I would wash my face and reapply it so that Carey never saw me make up free. I was convinced that if she saw me without make up she would make fun of me for being so ugly. Carey knew I wore it, it was not my secret anymore and she always teased me about it, but it was not so much of an issue to me now. I even went swimming during the holiday, though made sure that my face did not go under. I still panicked when it rained.

My face looked fine. I covered my nose with a thin layer of make up anyway, just to make sure and then I made my way to the gazebo.

Carey had chosen the music she wanted played as she walked down the aisle and I had no say in it. I had no say in much anymore and had got used to doing whatever pleased her. She wanted a pop song that had only just been in the charts and would no doubt be forgotten in a few more weeks. Its lyrics sang 'I've finally found what I'm looking for'. I guessed that Carey really believed it at the time. I wondered how she felt to be getting married. I wondered if I really was what she was looking for or whether she was just settling. I wondered if it was a big deal to her or, like me, it was just happening.

As the music played I stood at the gazebo staring ahead, looking back only now and again to see if Carey was there. I didn't know if I was supposed to look, I stood still and felt the emotion welling up inside. I didn't know what the emotion was; just that it was there in my gut and was pushing at my tear ducts. I felt helpless. I felt overwhelmed and then she was there, walking towards me, crying. Her dress had a red skirt that came up in a kind of an 'A' shape at the front; the top was a white P.V.C. corset. Her hair was blonde (as it had been for a while) and she wore a tiara. This was the girl I was going to marry and for some reason she wanted to marry me. Perhaps after this everything would be ok. Perhaps we could forget all that had happened in the past and move on as man and wife together. Perhaps this really was for the best.

I got carried away with the whole thing. I felt like crying but kept the tears away as I watched her walk up to me. She did look quite beautiful. She looked like a bride. I took her hand and smiled and we went up the steps to take our vows.

I don't know what those vows meant to Carey. I don't know if she really wanted me to be her husband. I don't know if she just saw me as someone that would look after her. What we fell in love for years before had all changed quite some time ago. I was marrying a sister that I hardly knew and she was marrying her dad. Together we could be ok, but it wasn't love, not really. We were at odds with each other. I was under her thumb. I was frightened to speak; afraid to be myself as I was told so many times that he was stupid. Despite this, there I was swearing to spend a lifetime like this, and there I was smiling for photographs and kissing her when the photographer asked us to, the first kisses we had shared in months.

After the ceremony and the photographs we sat with our feet in the swimming pool and we chatted about how it all went. I can't lie; I know we were happy, yet part of me wants to say we weren't. Part of me wants to think that I had some kind of foresight but that was what I definitely didn't have. I was going into this with blinkers on and I really thought it was all for the best. I didn't think things could be better. I didn't think I deserved anything better. Carey was now my wife.

It rained for the rest of the day and we played Scrabble with my mother and Nan under the shelter of the restaurant. Carey won. That was something that really annoyed me - the fact that I was the writer, I was the one that liked words yet Carey seemed to be able to beat me every time. I wasn't at all competitive, as a rule but that just seemed wrong some how. Anyway, that was about as romantic as it got. Playing Scrabble while we watched the rain. Perhaps the weather was trying to tell us something, but all I thought at the time was "Thank God it waited until after the wedding".

That night we watched a show put on as very questionable entertainment and left early. This was our wedding night after all and we hadn't been alone since the ceremony. In our room there was an ice bucket and a bottle of sparkling wine with two glasses. I opened it and poured it out while Carey squeezed herself out of her clothes.

"Turn around", she ordered. I was stunned at first, not sure what she had just said. "Turn around..." I couldn't believe it. Did I expect that things might be different now? Was it too much for her to have me see her body? She put on a nightshirt and I took my hand back away from my eyes. We drank the wine without a toast.

"I hope you don't think I'm going to sleep with you now that we're married?" Heaven forbid that I might have some strange delusion that we would be a normal married couple.

I could have had the marriage annulled but two years of celibacy and misery came before the inevitable divorce. Did I really believe that our marriage could be successful? What was I really hoping to achieve? Why did I see our lack of sex as a self-sacrificing purity? Why did I want so badly to be pure anyway? I thought that perhaps without sex in our lives there was one less thing to argue about. I thought that we alone had the key to a happy relationship. I thought we were better than other people who put so much store to physical love, but who was I trying to kid? I was human. I was a man. I had urges yet kept them away from my wife and away from myself. I swore that I would be pure and as for Carey I just presumed that she was not interested in sex at all. Our wedding day was the last time we ever kissed.

94

After the wedding we moved house and I moved jobs and worked for Oaklands, a higher paid job doing the same kind of work. I hated it there immediately. I hated the men with their sexual jokes and their constant farting. They seemed to think they were funny but it was all a bit of a culture shock to me. They would talk about pornography and women all the time and I just wanted to say that I thought they were all sick weirdos who needed to grow up and learn some respect. I was still a purest and I wanted them to know that I didn't approve, but that just made me an outcast. For the first six months or so I did not speak to anyone. How could I join in when I was a twenty five year old married virgin who hated his own sexuality? How could a sensitive man like me work in such a ladish environment?

I wanted to die. I really thought that if I had to spend my time with these people for five days a week, eight till five-thirty I would go insane. I didn't want this to be my life. Living with Carey with no love. Being dragged down by her, being told I was stupid, told I was wrong, told I was nothing. For the first time in years I really believed that I would have to end my life. I didn't know how it could change and I didn't think that I would ever be happy. I began to plan my death, planning when I might do it. I set a date and made a mark on the calendar. However, I had one problem - I was with someone now and my death would not just affect me this time, it would affect her as well.

I tried to put feelings of suicide aside and in time I became nullified to the guys at work. They were not all as bad as first impressions suggested, but I would never be like them and never wanted to be. They accepted that there was someone working there that was a little different and they grew to like me. I had stuck to my guns. As time went on I began to settle down at the place. I became good friends with Michael, a guy around my age that liked similar music to myself, and together we made it through each day chatting and having a laugh together. A year past, I got better at the job and moved up in the company a little. I actually began to enjoy working there. I enjoyed the time away from Carey and at work I could really be myself. No one there picked fault with my character or my clothes and there I could listen to the music that Michael and I liked, but Carey hated. We listened to The Smiths while we worked and sang along to the lyrics. 'Heaven Knows I'm Miserable Now.'

Then something disastrous happened.

Carey lost her job and she asked me to have a word with my boss about having her work with us. I tried to put her off by telling her what the men were like. I really didn't want her having to hear their lewd comments and I didn't want her invading my territory. But I couldn't tell her that, and she was out of work. I had no argument. I spoke to my boss and he agreed to have Carey there. So began the slow downward spiral that led to the death of my marriage.

Carey didn't seem phased by all the men at work and she took to the job just fine, but I was a joke to her, especially because I was technically above her. She wouldn't do anything I asked and she would laugh about me with the other guys. She seemed to be getting very chatty with a few of them and I wondered what she was saying. It was very awkward having her there, especially as we didn't really get on that well anymore. I avoided her as best I could and began to withdraw back into myself. I became quiet for I had to watch everything I said. The job began to get me down again.

Things just got worse between Carey and me. As the months went on anything we did still have in common fell apart. Carey was constantly on at me to change. Anything I tried to get into was a waste of time to her. Any music I liked was wrong. Any conversations we had were on a single and shallow wavelength. She seemed to only be interested in clothes, dance music and going to Stevenage's God awful nightclubs. I hated them; I would have rather died than go

96

there. I hated mixing with those people all there for a night of booze and dancing in that horrible mating dance that men did, grinding their bodies against the object of tonight's desire. I hated the loud depthless 'music' that had the same monotonous beat thumping through it like a heart all night, and even the alcohol didn't interest me. I had stopped getting drunk in public since I very nearly gave myself alcoholic poisoning some months before and narrowly escaped getting beaten up. There was nothing for me at those clubs and all I could think about was how suicide would get me out of all this once and for all. I thought that I could jump off the balcony and come crashing down onto the dance floor.

The only outlet I had for these feelings was my writing. I could never tell Carey the things that were going on in my mind but I could write them in my book. The main character in my novel became an enhanced version of me, depressed and hating his humanity. I got into his mind and I wrote about our feelings. 'Everyone has something in their lives they want to escape from, something in their past that has soured their taste for life, some have more than others....'

Carey didn't care that I hated going to those clubs and I made it no secret. I dreaded every weekend afraid that she would make us go there. I longed for her to meet some friends at work that she could go with. I wanted her to leave me alone. Well, as time went on we had some temporary staff in and she did become friendly with one of them. Now she would go out with her at the weekend and leave me behind to do whatever I wanted. I began to look forward to the times when I could be alone to write or read or do anything that had some depth to it. When she started to go out more often I did not think anything of it, I just enjoyed the space.

Outside of work I hated my life and inside of work my life was being sucked up by Carey's presence. I was

97

deeply unhappy. I remember New Year's night 1999. Everyone was planning their millennium celebrations and I was dreading it. I hated new years at the best of times but this was going to be the worst one. I hated that you had to celebrate it and you had to have such a great time. I hated being forced into enjoying myself and why should I be suddenly happy just because it was the 31st of December? I guess we celebrate that the year is going so that we can forget all the bad things that had happened and welcome in the new. But just because the date changes, doesn't mean that anything else will change. I was still married to a stranger and I still hated my life. I can't remember ever having a good New Year.

We went to my sister's that night along with my mother. We listened to music overly loud and had a few beers chatting, singing, playing with my two nieces. All should have been fine, but new years makes you think doesn't it? It is a time to think and re-evaluate your life, and mine was nothing but depressing. I had tried to join in the festivities but now my mind was taking over and everything just came piling in on me. My marriage was a farce. My job was a nightmare. I didn't get on with Carey anymore and just wanted to be left alone.

So I left the party. I guess that everyone thought I was just going in to the kitchen to get another beer but I kept going, straight out of the back door and away. I didn't know where I was going; I just wanted to be out of it, I just didn't want to pretend anymore. I think I could have easily killed myself that night. Part of me wanted to go to the train station and jump in front of a train. Part of me just wanted to hide, curl up in a ball and let the world drift by without my participation.

I just kept on walking, the night keeping me company, the stars lighting my way. I walked up into the town and stared into the shop windows, seeing myself reflected in the glass, a person I hardly knew anymore. I wanted to be me again.

As I wandered I heard fireworks going off in different places, everyone everywhere was having a party and here was I, about as low as I ever was, without hope and with no desire to live whatsoever.

My sister suddenly appeared beside me.

"What's the matter Steve? You scared us all."

"Sorry. I just can't do partying tonight. I have nothing to celebrate."

"You have all of us, you have Carey."

I wanted to spill my guts, tell all, let my sister know what a joke my marriage was, how Carey had no respect for me and made my life hell, but I didn't say any of that.

"I just don't want to be here."

"I know, I feel like that a lot of the time but I have the kids to look after and a husband. You just have to live for those things don't you?", but I didn't have those things.

She meant well, she talked me round, but deep in the core of myself I was broken for good. I went back to the party feeling just as suicidal but trapped in my body. My sister would not just stand by and let me do it, and with Carey around me all the time, suicide was never very practical but it was my dream, my ambition. All I wanted out of life was death.

As things got worse between Carey and me even when she was at home I did not see much of her. She said it was because she was with me all day at work that she didn't need to see me in the evenings. She would go up to the bedroom and tell me to stay downstairs. She had been getting interested in witchcraft and she said that she was doing spells up there. I wondered what sort of spells she might be doing. I wondered if any of them had anything to do with me, but I didn't have much of a worry about that. I was so unimportant in her life that I doubt she would waste her energies on me.

I knew that our relationship was as good as over. She would go out at strange times and answer text messages secretly. She would never tell me who they were from or where she was going. She said she was just going out to think and for some strange reason I believed her. I thought that although we hadn't got much in our relationship, we had got one thing, we had trust.

It would seem not.

We really did have to talk yet we never did anymore, so one Sunday afternoon I said that I wanted to go to the pub for a discussion and she agreed to come. It was a sunny day, although not that warm, and we sat on a bench in the pub garden. There was a pond there that I remembered having ducks on it but there were none at all today. We sat and for the first time in weeks we actually looked at each other and she smiled as if this was funny. I was deadly serious. I was ready to talk.

"Things have been getting bad between us for ages. I think we should have some time apart."

"Ok."

"You could live with your parents for a while."

"Right."

"Then maybe we could meet up sometimes, like have a date, like it used to be when we first met."

"Well... I think we should split up too. I'll move out."

She could have gone to her parent's house straight away but she didn't. She said that she didn't want to live with her parents at all and that she would get a flat with her friend from work. Apparently, the girl from work was just splitting up with her boyfriend and was looking for a flat mate. It was all falling into place for Carey, just like it always did.

Every night I had to sleep in the same bed as that girl that was still my wife but who happily wanted nothing to do with me. Sleeping right at the edge lest we have an awkward moment where our bodies touched, and we still worked together, don't forget that. I had to see her all day at work and then put up with her spending the evening in our bedroom casting spells with scented candles. I had been ousted. I was no longer part of my wife's life and she seemed perfectly ok about it. She was always cold about the whole thing, just as she was about everything. I wondered how we had come to this. I wondered when the exact moment was that we stopped loving each other.

I knew that it was my decision but it didn't feel like it. I had discussed a period of separation yet here she was planning her new life. She would rent a flat with this girl taking all her stuff with her. We were splitting up for real, but I wanted it. By then I was sick of my life and I wanted it back. I wanted myself back. I had got lost on the way, lost in the years of living for someone else. As soon as Carey was out of my hair I could start to live again. Perhaps it would all be for the best. Perhaps I could finish my book and get published and have a life with substance, but I wasn't interested in women. I vowed to myself right then that I would live like Morrissey; celibate and free of relationships. Because I obviously didn't adapt well to having a partner, I would be better off alone.

So it was met with some excitement when Carey eventually moved out. We argued over what she was going to take and what was mine and therefore had to stay. The fact was that it was my money that had bought most of our stuff, but I had to let her take some of it. She took the TV because her parents had given us it. She took the stereo, which I wasn't that bothered about because it had begun to go wrong anyway. She took her CDs (thankfully) and she took Hole's 'Celebrity Skin' which I quickly taped before I let her box it up. I closely guarded my CD collection and only let her have that one after much debate. I helped her pack and helped her carry out the stuff to the van. Jude from work was there. He was driving the van for them. He was getting very friendly with Carey I noticed and that annoyed me too. He helped lift out the three seater sofa and she left me the two seater. That was fine, I wasn't planning on entertaining. She took her books, and then she left. All three of them drove away and left me in the house alone to survey the damage.

It seemed that I had got off quite lightly. I still had the bed. I had a sofa. I had the furniture and most of the ornaments. I had all my CDs, though nothing to play them on. I had the rabbit. I had my freedom.

A few purchases had to take place to make my bachelor pad fit my lifestyle. My mother gave me a lift to Stevenage and I went to the used computer shop there to buy a system. I had now finished my first novel and wanted to type it all out. I also wanted to get on the internet. There was a whole world out there and I wanted to be part of it. For far too long it had just been me and Carey and I had lived my life in blinkers. No more.

She had moved out and the computer came in. That and a desk and a new stereo and I was set up. I would live the dream I had been striving for. A life of peace and, I smiled as I thought of it, I would never have to go to a nightclub ever again.

The only problem I had now was that I still had to work with her. We had never argued much and we didn't really wish each other any ill, but seeing her every day was rubbing my nose in it a little. It would have probably been ok if it weren't for the growing friendship she was having with Jude. He was ten years older than her, had a kid and lived with his partner, and I never thought that there was anything blossoming between them. I was wrong. Carey kept it from me but I soon got it out of her.

"Are you seeing someone?" I asked while we stood together out in the lunch area.

"Yes."

"Is it Jude?"

The silence that followed was answer enough, but she wasn't going to leave it at that when she could happily dish out another spray of venom.

"Yes it's Jude."

"Were you seeing him while we were together?"

"No, but he has moved in the flat with us."

Great. What was I supposed to do now? Was I supposed to go into the warehouse and act as if I didn't know? Was I supposed to go in there and punch the guy's lights out? What he had done was dreadful; moving in on my wife as soon as she left my house, but she was the one to blame really wasn't she? It was her decision to do this. So I swallowed hard and I went on as if I didn't care, all the time believing that she had cheated on me, and feeling for the first time that it was really over. I didn't want her back. I wanted to be alone.

Solitude

I knew it was over between Carey and me, I also knew what 'over' meant, but I don't think that Carey did. Carey didn't want this to be the end of her and me; she wanted to be 'friends'. Friends with this girl that had dragged me half way across the world to make pointless vows to someone she was supposed to love and then spent the next two years trying to change him. She even told me at some stage that she wanted the old Steve back; the one I had been when we first met. I could have strangled her! It was her that had forced me to change! It was for her that I was wearing a bloody green T-shirt. Well I was going to change right back, be myself, and be alone. The coloured T-shirts could all go to charity and I would wear the black ones again. I would even take a trip to Camden at some stage and do some shopping in the markets. I was already enjoying this new found freedom and I could do well without Carey hanging around me like a bad smell.

When I first got my computer I spent weeks sifting through the scribbling that were my first novel, piecing it all together. There were yellow highlighted parts here and red crossed bits there. There were asterix, arrows, footnotes and post-its with lines on. Some of the pages were written on the back, some were not. Pages were numbered but then there were extra pages marked, for example, 6B, to include late additions to the text. It was a mess, but I devoted all my spare time to it, locking my door and sitting at my desk for hours and hours, drinking cider as I worked. There was nothing to disturb me. That was until I got the internet.

I didn't go online for a good few weeks but when I finally did, I was very excited and spent hour after sapping hour on the damn thing. Straight away I was on there discovering things about the music I loved, visiting official web sites and fan sites and then there was the discovery of forums and chat rooms. There was a whole world out there! And no one was looking over my shoulder telling me not to look up when Tori Amos's new album was coming out or where I could get hold of her rare CD singles. No one was telling me that I was an obsessed fan just because I joined the discussion forum and posted a few answers to people's posts telling them my favourite songs off 'Boys For Pele'. No one was going to stop me going on Ebay and bidding on a Living Dead Doll. No one would poke fun at me for buying this girlfriend substitute, a little gothic friend to share my desk with me. That was one of the first things I bought on there but certainly not the last. My money was my money now and there is nothing better to fill a hole in your life than buying stuff.

After the initial excitement of being connected to the wide world of computer nerds I continued with my novel. It was coming along nicely and was all making so much more sense now that it was typed out. Half way through a page I would suddenly think of something I wanted to know or something I wanted to buy and I would go online for a while. It was a constant distraction but thankfully my only one. I hadn't really got any friends left, I would only see my family occasionally, I was wrapped up in my own little world and I was fine.

However, Carey wouldn't leave me alone. She would phone me and tell me how her life was going as if I really cared. She would talk to me at work as if everything was ok. Well it wasn't ok. She had treated me terribly and had left me for another man. I didn't care if things between Carey and Jude were going well or if they weren't. I could have done without any damn contact from her at all, but she would ring late at night and talk to me for hours then say she was only calling to arrange coming over to pick up more stuff. She would come over after work in Jude's car and take another box full of things that we would have to argue about. She kept me on the end of her strings and I couldn't move on, I couldn't have the breathing space to really think. It took six months for the failure of my marriage to finally hit me.

One phone call I wasn't expecting, mere weeks into the separation, was to begin my grieving process.

"Steve."

"Carey." I wanted to say, "What do you want". I wanted to be harsh, but I never was.

"I want you to sort out us getting a divorce."

A divorce? This was supposed to be a trial separation! She had given it three weeks and she was asking for a divorce! It sounded so strange, so surreal. I was too young to be getting a divorce. Could this really be my life?

"Oh." I couldn't hide my shock.

"Well we may as well. We're not getting back together are we?"

I guess there never was a chance that we would get back together, it had gone too far, but this still seemed a little extreme.

"What's the rush?"

"I just want it sorted out. I don't want to get married again or anything I just want to clear things up. And I want to come over and borrow the photographs. I'll look through them and take what I want then give them back."

"Ok. Well how do I sort out a divorce?"

"Have a look online. I don't know. I'll come after work tomorrow."

"What?"

"For the photos."

And that was it. So now I did have something to use the internet for. At age twenty-six here I was looking up sites about divorces and how you put it all in process. It was scarily easy. You could even download the paperwork, if you paid for it. When Carey came over the next evening I told her what I had found and she told me to go ahead and download the forms. She really did want this and she wanted it now. She would give me half the money and we would get together to fill them in. So began my divorce proceedings.

I downloaded the forms and printed them out and Carey and I spoke at work about when we would fill them in together. I couldn't stop thinking about the idea of getting our marriage annulled. I wondered if it was still part of the law that you consummate your marriage. I spent some time thinking on whether I would prefer to do that than go through these court proceedings, but how could I prove that we had never had sex? Who would believe me in this day and age? I could hardly believe it myself. I didn't really want to admit it to anyone. So a divorce it was, but on what grounds? I read the forms and saw that you had to have a legitimate reason to dissolve the marriage. This was the first thing I asked Carey.

"I'll say that I cheated on you." She suggested.

It sounded so cold, so without regret. I wondered why she found this so easy.   "Did you?"

"No. You know I didn't. I didn't start seeing Jude until we had split."

I didn't know if I believed her. Why would she want it on record that she had done that if she hadn't? I guess it didn't matter. It was her decision and if she admitted to infidelity the divorce would, no doubt, go through quickly. Let her get on with it then. Let her do this if she wanted a divorce so badly. At least she hadn't suggested that I say it was me that cheated - that would be more like one of her tricks. We filled the forms in - lying about dates that she started seeing this 'other man', but all the time I was thinking - she did start going out a lot, on her own, she could have been seeing him. She probably was and I was probably stupid for not realising. I had trusted her, but I didn't trust anything she said anymore.

It took hours to fill the forms in and being with Carey for so long was quite uncomfortable. There was nothing between us anymore, no love, and no attraction. She was even taking the 'mickey' out of me for the pain behind my eyes, because for her this was easy. I realised for the first time, now that we were officially apart, just how evil and damaging she really was. The divorce was for the best because the marriage should never have happened. Once this was done I didn't have to have anything more to do with her.

She had brought the photographs back and once she had left I sat and looked through some of them. We used to take a lot of photos; I guess we were just vain. I always looked so much better in pictures than I looked in real life. If people only saw the pictures they would probably think I was good looking. There were a lot of pictures of Carey that she had not taken for herself. Photos taken in the first couple of years when our relationship still meant something. I looked at them and felt sad. I was sad that it had come to this, wondering how something good could end up so twisted. She was a different person in those photos. I didn't really know her anymore and if I had met her now, I would not have been interested in her. We had nothing in common now. We had different minds. I put the photos away and put them back in a drawer in the bedroom. I guessed that I would always keep them because they were still part of my life, but I probably wouldn't look at them again.

The next day, at work, I asked Carey if she had taken all the photos she wanted, as there didn't appear to be many missing. She looked at me with a smirk and said:

"Well I didn't want any of you."

Was she trying to hurt me as much as possible? Splitting up was painful enough without straight away living with another man, without constantly calling me and coming over to take more stuff. Then she said that and my faith in her just shattered. There was truly nothing left that she could do to me. I wondered if she had always been like this or whether she had just grown up to be this mega bitch. My family had always had their doubts about her; they had always made it quite clear that they didn't think she was a very nice person. How come I was the last to know? What had I seen in her that they hadn't, and was it all just an illusion? Perhaps I was just a terrible judge of character because this was the real Carey, the Carey that no longer had to care about my feelings. This was Carey in the raw, and now it was all too clear that we should not, and probably should never, have been together.

I finished typing up my book, printed it all out and was ready to send it off to publishers. I was quite pleased with it, and should have been considering I had been writing the damn thing for five years. It had been subjected to two complete rewrites and then a lot of jiggling around once it was put on computer and now, at last, it was completed. 'Personal Demons', the book I just had to write, the book that told a story of my own inner anguish with depression and suicidal urges. A novel filled with views on life and after life. It was my first novel. Twenty-six years of life and I had finally achieved something. I was quite proud of myself.

I went to the library and sat with the 'Writers and Artists Year Book' copying addresses of potential publishing houses. I was planning to send it away to quite a few different places, but I had to be careful to only send it to those that published my kind of book. The trouble was I didn't really know what 'my kind of book' was. It was about madness and about the after life, but it was not really a horror story or a crime novel or anything else that they categorised. I just had to take some chances.

I enjoyed sitting there working on my writing career. I felt intellectual and felt that I was the Stephen I wanted to be. I guess I was filled with hope at that stage. I truly believed that my novel could get published and my life could turn around. I would have something to live for. I could quit work and my writing would be my new job. I could sit at home and write, not having to cope with seeing people, not having to put on my public face. I would get acclaim and money, and I could keep on writing and get those books published as well. Then I wouldn't care about Carey and she would be sorry that she had thrown away a relationship with a published author.

As the rejections came pouring in those hopes began to seem like fantasies. Who was I to think that I could be anything? Obviously my writing was useless and I never would get published because I just didn't deserve to. If only

I could get one positive response. I knew that it was a difficult novel. I knew that it was depressing to read, but that was the whole idea! Art is made to get a reaction, it doesn't really matter what that reaction is. It used to matter. Art used to be defined as something that was pleasant, but that wasn't true anymore. My book was art!

I took the old pages of my novel, the hand written copies with their highlights and their arrows and I stood on my bed and began to blue-tac them to the walls. This was art. Writing as art, art of writing. I chose the most poignant pages; my favourite passages and I stuck each page side by side around the room. I was hiding the horrible floral border that ran around just under the ceiling and at the same time making a statement. I always felt that I had to make statements.

The next statement I made was another tattoo. The divorce was going through and I needed to say something about it, make a lasting declaration that this was not the end for me. I chose some writing, a comment that I was a writer myself, and I chose the lyrics from a Tori Amos song. I chose the words 'Little Earthquakes'. In that song she sings, "give me life, give me pain, give me my self again." That said what I wanted to say. These things that have happened to me were just little earthquakes and I could learn from them and move on, rebuild, and the fact that Carey couldn't stand Tori Amos, just made it all the more significant. It was her fault I had got into Tori Amos in the first place. She had one song by her on a mix tape and I always liked it and asked her who it was. Then Carey did what was probably the nicest thing she had ever done and probably the best thing she ever did for me. She bought me a Tori Amos album. From that moment Tori Amos was my confidant. She got me through some real dark times and was a real friend to me. When I was still with Carey I would sit listening to her music on my personal stereo and go completely in to her world. It was where I liked to escape to, but now that I was single I could actually live there. I got the tattoo done on my lower back and the pain (of which was the worst pain of all my tattoos) just made it all the more poignant.   I didn't want Carey to know about the tattoo so I didn't tell anyone at work. That tattoo was mine and mine alone. It was my secret, although I did go online and tell everyone on the Tori Amos forum. I got a lot of replies to my message saying how cool it was.

It was getting hard for me to keep sane with everything that was around me. I still had to face Carey and Jude every day at work and they were always together laughing and mucking around. They had no respect for my feelings at all and I don't know how I kept composed. All the guys there were on my side and when they could get me on my own for a few minutes, they would say how they had never really liked Carey and that I was better off alone.

I had the divorce to contend with as well, although that seemed to be going through without any problems. I just wanted shot of it all now. I wanted Carey out of the way, but I never told her. I was never anything but polite. She would still talk to me at work as though we were friends that just happened to have spent seven years together and life was fine and going on, as it should. However, this was not a normal situation and not one that I could really cope with. I was filled with bitterness and I hated Jude.

After months of living like this there was a meeting called at work and we all stopped what we were doing and looked round to see my boss, Carey and Jude all standing together.

"Right everyone," my boss said, "Jude and Carey have been to see me this morning and they have announced that they are leaving us. They will work out the week. I'm sure we all wish them well in whatever they do. Thanks."

There were mumblings and whispers but I knew what they were saying. They were all pleased that the bad element was to be removed. Things would run a lot more smoothly and I, they guessed, would be a lot happier.

I didn't know how I felt. I was as good as divorced from a girl I had known for seven years and now she was to leave my life completely. It would be weird not seeing that face, but it surely had to be for the best. Now I could get on with my life.

…But I had no life to get on with. I hated my job, even with Carey gone; I still didn't like having to go there each day pretending I was ok. I was completely alone in my one bed house, single again at twenty-six. I didn't know how to be single again. I didn't know how to be happy alone and I didn't know how to find anyone else. Carey had scared away all my friends and my family had their own lives. Six months of solitude and the truth of my split from Carey finally hit me. Six months of being single that I had coped with, but now I was falling and falling hard. All the bad feelings I had ever had came back times three; feelings of utter loneliness and hopelessness. I was free falling down the pit of despair. I couldn't see out of it, couldn't even see that there was a way out. I was living a life with nothing. Nothing I used to enjoy was giving me any pleasure. I was constantly feeling depressed and wanting to die. I had no one to help me. I had no drugs to help me and I wouldn't accept any help. My mother and sister would ask to see me and I would say that I wanted to be alone. I wanted to write, I wanted to hide my face, but the solitude was eating into my brain.

I was cutting myself again. Cutting so that I could feel something real. Cutting to get over the urge to die. Cutting myself to see if I had the courage it would take to slit my wrists. I would break open a razor and take the thin sharp metal strips out, and then I would do it, slowly at first, feeling the stinging pain…A couple of cuts on my inner wrist, over the light blue veins that I could see under my pale skin.

114

How deep would I have to cut to sever them and see my life flood out? Did I have what it takes to do that…to push hard and run the blade through the veins? After a few times the pain numbed and I did it quickly and heavier, slashing my arm, the blood coming freely. My wrist would be a wash with red and I would keep doing it, getting out the aggression that I had, the anger I had about having to be alive.

I remembered those times that I had decided to die and how I used to make dates, now I wrote a computer diary and I set a date once more. Every day I wrote of my misery, of my utter urge to die. I wrote about having nothing in my life to live for. I wrote about hating everything that was human; relationships, working, futile entertainments, socialising, and going to the God damn toilet.   I hated it all. I hated the whole human condition. I wrote pages about how my skin was disgusting and about how it hindered my life. It was getting as bad as it used to be when I worked at the hospital. More and more I was getting obsessed with my appearance. While with Carey the problem I had with my face had never completely gone away, but it had certainly been better.   Now it had started to hinder me again. Stopping me from functioning and living a normal life.

I would only shave at night and in the dark, and luckily I didn't need to shave every day. I would try and put it off but I didn't like facial hair and mine would grow in random sprouts here and there - it had to go. I had the light on in the landing so that I could just about see what I was doing but didn't have a bright view of my skin. I couldn't bear to look at my face without make up; it scared me, repulsed me and made me start to panic. The last thing I wanted to see while shaving was my own red nose and cheeks.

Once I had finished shaving I would dry my face on the towel and go into the bedroom holding the towel to my face. There was a full-length mirror in there and the light was a little kinder than the light in the bathroom. In the bedroom I dared to slowly move the towel from my face and stare at my reflection. I would get really close and move my face at different angles to check every millimeter of skin. The overall appearance, I believed, was of someone with bad skin, but close up I could focus on each separate part and try to improve it. I would pick at spots and get rid of them, but usually my tampering would leave a mark bigger than the spot ever was. I got my nails deep into my skin trying to gouge out any trace of the spot, leaving myself with little bloody wounds. Then there were the marks I had made last time, scabs on my skin that I picked off when they were not ready to go. There was always something going on with my face, healing in process that I would never allow to show.

My skin was too thin, that's what I decided. My outer layer of skin was thin and you could see the blood vessels inside of it. I had squeezed my nose until it was red to get all the puss out but now it was red and I could not bear to look at it. It was always red; the blood pumping around it was visible and ugly. I needed to grow new skin. I put a layer of Savlon over it hoping it would encourage new skin to grow while I slept. Perhaps I would wake up the next day and it would be repaired, but it never was.

Shaving often missed bristles that were growing like black heads under the surface. They could not be allowed to stay. I went into the bathroom to get the tweezers and came back determined to clear my face of those hideous black hairs. With my face pressed against the glass I put the tweezers against my skin and attempted to get hold of the tiny black bristles. I would try for ages sometimes, missing it with every attempt, getting panicky that I wouldn't be able to get rid of it, pushing the tweezers harder against my flesh. More often than not I would get the hair but leave a wound on my skin where I had been pressing the metal against myself. Another mark to ruin the overall picture of my skin, spots, cuts, scabs and dry skin. I started to freak out, scared that I might be seen like this, afraid that the door would knock, afraid that I would not be able to get to work the next day.

116

I put more Savlon over the fresh wounds and all over my thin skin and then I went to bed. Lying on my back so that the cream didn't rub off on my pillow and so that the air could get to my wounds. This was a ritual I had begun to perform every night and every night I would be reduced to tears because I was so ugly, so trapped in such hideous skin, and everyone would see, everyone would see this monstrous aberration. I begged for it to get better, for the next day to not be impossible. For if I couldn't get my skin to look something close to normal how could my work colleagues see me? All those eyes staring at Steve, thinking how ugly he is, how gross he looked. I wished that death would take me in my sleep, but I didn't even want anyone to see me looking like this when I was dead. Sometimes I would put make up on before I went to bed, worried that there might be a fire and I would have to leave the house without any on. Worried that if I died in the night my body would have to be identified looking red and covered in sores. However, usually I would try to keep my face free of make up when no one was there to see, because I truly believed that I had to have new skin grow and it couldn't grow over make up. I tried to give my skin a rest over night in the hope that I would wake up normal.

I lay in bed, afraid to move, feeling my skin with the tips of my fingers. I felt for more missed bristles, for any new spots. I sometimes felt something and had to get up to check it or to start the whole process again. Sometimes I would lie in bed trying to pull facial hair out with my fingers. I would try again and again to grab hold of the bristle and pull it free of my skin. Sometimes I would manage it and feel a real sense of achievement, other times I would just stay awake for hours picking and picking. Sometimes I had a spot that I had squeezed and the skin was swollen. I would lay there with my finger pressed hard against it believing that if I squashed the skin down for long enough the swelling would go down, though it never did.

I kept a mirror in my bedside cabinet and I would take it out to look at myself again. I would lay there holding the mirror at arms length, looking much better in the moonlight, my skin grey and the blemishes dulled. I would put the lamp on but the bulb was red and that made me look almost flawless. I liked to look at myself with the red light on and try to convince myself that I really looked that good, that I was really quite good looking, not a monster at all, but who was I trying to kid?

I woke each morning to the shrill cry of the alarm clock and a lump would form in my throat, a lump of fear, of utter dread. I wanted it to be a bad dream. Surely I could not look as bad as I thought? Surely last night was not normal; I would look better in the light of day. I would reach for the mirror and I would start with it close up against my nose, looking at myself, slowly moving it away to give myself a true image. Were there any fresh spots? Were the wounds healed? Had that swollen pore gone down? And every time, I looked worse than I had ever imagined and I put the mirror back in the cabinet with the hope that I would look better in the bathroom mirror.

I couldn't lie in bed for any time because it would take me a good hour to sort out my skin. I knew the routine but sometimes things just wouldn't go to plan. I would wash my face and put on the make up, over my nose first, then any other areas that looked red or had spots. I thought that the area under my lips was particularly bad; the skin there was really thin and so I would cover it. Then check what I looked like in the shaving mirror, held up against the window so that I could see my face in daylight. That was the real test. Doing that often exposed new areas to sort out and proved whether or not I had made the make up look natural. The day light test was harsh and I always dreaded it, but if I looked ok in daylight then I was ready for work. An hour of panic, of working hard to make myself acceptable, of looking in all the different mirrors in my house, and then it would be eight o'clock and I was already late.

I would think that I had finished sorting my face out and I would put my coat and shoes on, then I would take what I promised to be just one last look at myself in the living room mirror. Then it would all go wrong. Did I really look that awful? I would see something I missed, see a little bit of flaking skin I hadn't removed or a bristle of facial hair I hadn't plucked and I would run back up to the bathroom to sort it out. It would be gone eight now, time I should be at work, but I resigned myself to the fact that I would be late. Then I would see more things and I would get panicky at the thought of people seeing me in such a state. My heart would race and my breathing would come in fits. I couldn't go in to work looking like this. My nose would be redder than I thought and there would be peeling skin on it. I looked like a freak.

I would look at my watch and see that it was now quarter past, the people at work would have started to talk, started to ask the question "where is Steve?" But how could I go in with a nose like that? I could probably make it in for half past. I would wash my nose and scrub it with a sponge, but then it would be bright red and it would take a good half an hour to get it back to an acceptable state. I would put Savlon on it first for a smoother surface, then the make up. I could taste my breath; feel the blood pumping too fast around my body. The time would be ticking and I would be getting more and more scared. Afraid that people will see me before I am ready, scared that I will lose my job. I would turn up at work at quarter to nine and say that I over slept. I 'over slept' a lot.

Other times it would be worse. Perhaps there would be one spot on my face that was so prominent that it made my whole face distorted. Perhaps I just couldn't sort out my nose. I would panic and I would try to calm my breathing, staring into the shaving mirror, close to tears as I saw my skin in daylight. I would run from room to room looking in different mirrors and anything reflective praying that it wasn't true, that I didn't really look like that. Then I would break down completely. I just couldn't do it, my face was just too hideous, and if I couldn't sort it out by around nine o' clock then I just wouldn't go in to work at all. I would wash all the make up off, cover it in Savlon and go and lie in my room for the day. I would text my boss at work and tell him I was ill, which was basically true. Two hours of working on my face, panicking and concentrating would make me physically sick. My boss didn't know anything about my mental health. I don't know what they thought with my constant lateness and with all those random days away.

How could I live like this? How could I live when I despised myself? How could I live in their world when I looked like a monster? How could I live in a world I wanted no part of? How could I live now that my hope had gone? My hope for a better life was being shattered daily. I had sent so many samples of my book to publishers that I got a rejection slip nearly every day. If it weren't for the Tori Amos CDs I kept receiving from Ebay, I would have dreaded the postman. One day the post brought me a different kind of news. It was news that the divorce was final.

I didn't know how I was supposed to react. I was in a daze for the whole day. Half of me was pleased, half of me was devastated. I told everyone at work and they all supported me, telling me it was a new start and a really good thing. Michael was there to cheer me up, to make me laugh, but this was really serious. I was a divorcee, I was single again, I was a virgin, I couldn't drive, my job was not well paid and had no prospects, I still felt depressed all of the time, I still wore make up because I was convinced I looked disgusting, and the only person that had put up with all this was gone. I couldn't take it for long.

I wrote my diary, pages embracing the idea of death, longing for it, yet something always held me back. The dates I set for my suicide came and went without any action. I kept finding reasons to put it off, saying that I would do it at the end of the month, putting it off until I had been to see

120

Tori Amos live…but soon I would run out of pathetic reasons to keep myself on Earth. Soon it would just get too much for me.

August 30th, Union chapel, Islington: The last thing I had been holding my death off for came and left within a couple of hours. I saw Tori Amos play a concert in a church. It was a religious experience, a touch of beauty in my world that longed for something to touch me. It touched me; the piano playing loud and dark or pretty and melodic, the songs with words reaching into my mind and soul. A soulful voice with bitter anguish or utter delight. I loved every second of it and I didn't want it to end for I knew this was it. I had gone with a work colleague and he asked if I had enjoyed it, well 'enjoy' wasn't a strong enough word. I had just been through something that had affected my every emotion. I had nearly cried as she sang the words to 'Icicle'…'I could have, I should have…' screamed with utter passion. I told him that I could now die happily. I knew what I meant.

It wasn't long after that before I broke down completely. I had stopped setting myself dates because I just didn't stick to it, but the thing I had been holding off for was over. I had no reason to keep living my life, if indeed I ever had. Holding off the date of my suicide for the sake of a concert, for a new CD release, for the chance that life would get better just seemed over optimistic. I had no optimism. I was in no doubt that my life was over. At work I opened up my Stanley knife and took out a fresh blade. I figured it would be better than the blade from a razor.

'Dear diary,

If I was to slit my wrists, you know, really slit them - not just the aesthetic interpretation I usually perform - what would it be like? I mean, the pain would be quick, the horror would last for hours, but the fascination is so great it seems worthwhile. Which vein do I need to sever? Which vein holds the most life to spill? …Life draining out into my bath and down the plug hole. Not romantic, but sick and sharp, yet still not such a bad way to leave. I need guts to cut deep. My cuts are mere scratches that embarrass and sting the next day. I will have to be brave for a moment, but bravery will only come when I am my most weak. I want to die; I want to want to die. I wish I wanted it enough. I hate life. I hate death. Sleep is nice, but is death like sleep? It doesn't seem like it is - it seems that it is more final than that. Will I wake and think, "That was nice, I think I'll have a lie in". Or will I never wake at all. Am I ready for that? When will I be?'

My mother came to my house on Sunday with the discs that contained her book. She had just finished her first novel too but had written it on a word processor. I thought that I might be able to convert them on my PC. I tried to be positive for her, but inside I was thinking, "What is the point? There's no way either of us are going to get published." I had not read my mother's work and she had not read mine. If even our own flesh and blood were not interested in reading them how could we expect a different reaction from a publisher? …But I didn't say any of this. I helped her out.

I found a program on the internet that would convert them but would cost ninety pounds. A trial version would convert the files but corrupt the text with spelling mistakes. I asked her...

"Shall I do it? Shall I press the button that will convert it all? Then you will have to go through it and correct everything."

"What do you think I should do?"

I had no answer. I had no interest. All I could think about was that I had work the next day and I looked awful. I wished that my mother wasn't there. I wished that I could hide away. I wondered what my mother thought when she looked at me. I wondered if she thought that I was ugly, a nice face spoilt by bad skin. Was that what everyone that saw me thought? "What a shame he would be such a nice looking lad if only it wasn't for his skin". I wondered if my mother knew that I wore make up. I had not told her. I had not told anyone.

"You need to have it on Word for a publisher, I say do it."

And I did it for her and saved the mess that was now her novel on to a floppy disc.

My mother stayed with me all afternoon talking about writing and then left me for the evening. Alone I felt no more comfortable, for I still had to see myself. I still hated looking in the mirror yet I could not stop myself, looking in one then looking in another begging for change. I washed the make up off in my dark bathroom and stood with my hands holding the sink as I stared long and hard into the mirror. There were cuts that wouldn't heal, cuts I had made myself but that didn't make it any better. I couldn't even cover them with make up, they were huge gaping, weeping sores. No way could I go to work looking like this and what were the chances of it getting better over night?

I took a bottle of cider upstairs and lay on my back in my bedroom, my eyes surveying my surroundings. I drank and I looked at the posters as they became slowly veiled in the waning light. I looked at all the pages of my novel stuck to the walls. Was I crazy? Was that a crazy thing to do and why had I bothered? Getting published was a pipe dream, as stupid an ambition as becoming a rock star or a film star.

It wasn't going to happen to me. Nothing good was ever going to happen to me.

I lay in the room looking around me until it had got too dark to see anything, and then I swung my legs over the side of the bed and sat upright thinking dark and twisted thoughts. I wanted to cut, that's what the matter was. I needed to get those scrambled feelings out of me. There was only one way to let out my inner anguish and that was to open my flesh. The drink was not enough this night, the kick I was getting from the usual cider was dull and forgotten. I went downstairs, turning on the landing light, and got to my black work bag. The blade I had stolen was in there, silver and freshly sharp, it seemed to offer me an answer, it seemed to be speaking to me. "Now is the time. There is no reason to put it off anymore. Tonight is the night".

I ran back up the stairs and into the bathroom, I didn't turn on the light. I knelt on the carpet floor with my arms over the bath and I looked at my white clean skin. I wouldn't be happy until they were a wash with red blood. I didn't deserve such clean arms. I didn't deserve to be alive. I picked up the shaving mirror and looked in to it, staring at my flawed complexion in the grey darkness. I hated that it was me. I hated myself. I hated life.

I put the mirror back away and I held out my right arm so that I was looking at the inner wrist. There were old scars there, thin red lines that would give me away if anyone were to see. They were my secret but my secret was about to be announced to the world. I took the Stanley blade and with hardly another thought I slashed at my arm. The blade must have been really sharp as the cut was quite deep and shocked me a little, but I had started now and I couldn't let the sight of my own ripped flesh put me off. I did it again, not being quite so harsh and I slashed and slashed until there were about five fresh cuts oozing blood. I had cut over the veins but the blood was only coming slowly, I had obviously not cut deep enough. I hated myself for being so weak, for not having the strength to open the veins, but I did have the strength I just hadn't used it yet. I cut a few more times over the lower part of my wrist, just where I thought you had to cut in order to die. I hardly felt the pain now, but yet again the blood merely leaked slowly out. The first cut had been the deepest and trickles of blood were running out of it and down my arm in a red trail. ...And so I aimed the blade at that cut, slashing myself in the exact same place so that it would go deeper into my skin. I did it and it hurt, I recoiled away hissing through clenched teeth "Shit, shit, shit," but it had worked. Blood started to drip from the wound drip after drip counting down second after second. I wondered if I had done enough, whether I could actually bleed to death. I wanted it so badly. I didn't want to have to go to work the next day, or any day. I didn't want to have to look at myself ever again. I didn't want to go through day after lonely day, night after lonely night, sleeping and waking up alone. I wanted this to be it.

I looked at my left arm, so far untouched by tonight's terrible events. I slashed at it viciously with the blade, trying to hold the weapon straight and tight with bloody fingers. I did it a few times and then I aimed higher, aiming for the same place that was dripping like a broken tap from my right arm. I slashed it and it opened deeply, then I slashed it again and again, cutting within the cut, the sharp pain making me wince, but it worked. Both arms were cut in the same place and both wounds were dripping blood, splashing down in my clean white bath.

I knelt there, leaning my weight against the bath as I watched the blood pour down both arms and then drip from my elbows. The whiteness of the bathroom was being splashed with red, dark and cathartic, life running out of me, all of my pain focused on watching myself die. ...But I felt nothing, no dizziness, no light-headedness, and although the blood was dripping fast it was only dripping, not gushing or spurting and I couldn't handle cutting anymore, it hurt too much, the whole idea was repugnant to me now. I was shaking from the pain and the shock and the trauma, but I liked watching myself bleed. I liked that I had caused myself such harm. I tried to believe that I had done it, that I had successfully slit my wrists and would soon enough die and be spared the horrors of the next day. …But the longer I knelt there the more it seemed apparent that I had not done enough, I was going to live.

The bath was black with blood and my arms were still dripping relentlessly but at this rate it would take me days to bleed to death, if indeed the wounds didn't just heal themselves. It was a sudden realisation that made me stand up and look at myself long and hard in the mirror with my arms still held out over the bath. I suddenly got a reality check. I was not going to die. This was another failed and pathetic attempt at my life.

I wrapped toilet paper round and round my arms and the blood started soaking through straight away. I wrapped more around them and slowly walked down the stairs, disappointed with what I was about to do, I was going to ring for an ambulance.

"Yes, I need an ambulance."

"Ok. Can you tell me what has happened?"

"I've slit my wrists."

"Ok, is the blood gushing out?"

No such luck.

"It's dripping fast."

"Ok, where are you?"

126

As soon as I had made the call I rushed back into the bathroom and turned on the light. The bath was a mess with splashes of blood all over it and a thick puddle of black just under where I had let my arms drip. ...But I had gone back in there for a reason, I had to put on my face; I needed to put on my make up.

With blood soaking through the tissue wrapped around my wrists I applied make up to my nose and to a number of other problem areas. I knew that I didn't have time to do a good job but I couldn't leave the house without some amount of camouflage. I did it quickly, not looking too close for I knew that it would not pass the usual tests, but I got myself ready to face the public. I was scared of what might happen to me at the hospital, but resigned to the fact that I had failed again and my arms would need sewing up.

I saw flashing blue lights through the window in my front door and I went outside to greet the paramedics. There was a young man with blonde hair and as he got nearer to me he looked a little taken aback yet I'm sure he had seen much worse than this.

"Where's the weapon?" He asked.

I had to think.

"In the bath."

"What did you use?"

"A Stanley blade."

"Ok we're going to take you in to the ambulance and get those wounds dressed up for you ok?"

I was feeling feeble, feeling scared and feeling dreadfully suicidal. I believe that I have lived with a feeling that I want to die for years, but to actually feel suicidal, to actually feel that you could in fact do it, is a terrible feeling. It is a rock in your chest, a pulling on your throat, and clouding of thought. It is tunnel vision, a shaking in your hands, and a dark fog in your mind. I needed to be looked after. I needed to be in hospital, warm and sterile, cleaned and made better. I was in a dark place, the bathroom was its shrine, but I wanted them to take me away from it. Perhaps that was all I had ever wanted.

In the back of the ambulance there was a female paramedic and she greeted me. I wondered what they were really thinking. They probably thought I was a freak. They took the sodden tissue away from my cuts and washed my arm. The biggest cut was still bleeding steadily. The female paramedic wiped it with cotton wool and seemed to be trying to look inside it, the blood came as soon as it was cleaned.

"Are these old cuts?"

"Some of them are old, some are from tonight." My voice was frail and I was shaking. The male paramedic wrapped a clean white dressing over the whole lower arm and then did the same with my left arm.

"What's your name?" He asked.

"Stephen."

I think he told me his name, I don't remember it now, but I was very thankful for his care. He didn't seem cross that I had done this to myself. I wondered if the nurses at hospital would be so understanding.

I felt each curve in the road as we made our way to hospital and once there I was rushed through and was sitting in front of a nurse right away. The blonde haired paramedic smiled back at me.

"Ok you'll be looked after now."

I thanked him and he left. For a few seconds I felt abandoned, but then the nurses took over. They walked me into a cubicle and pulled the curtains around me. There they unwrapped my arms and surveyed the damage, I was still bleeding.

"Ok we're going to have to try and stop the bleeding." The nurse said, "Hold your arm up. Have you had a tetanus booster lately?" I knew it had only been a few years since Carey's dog had bitten me on the nose; the scar was there to remind me.

"Yes, I had one a few years ago."

There seemed to be a lot of coming and going, a lot of nurses looking at my arm and then wrapping it back up. Time was going by yet I had no perception of it. I was in a daze, wishing I was dead; wishing they would not be able to mend me and that I would slowly bleed to death while they looked for a way to stop the blood. I wondered whether they had put me on low priority because they were dealing with other people, people that actually wanted saving. I was not in my right mind, I was in the suicide place, a dark oubliette, ostracised from my own sanity. Down in a deep dark hole where nurses would come and stare down occasionally calling down to me to see if I was still ok. Well, I wasn't ok. I was far from ok. Life was miserable yet death was harsh and hard to get to. I didn't know if I was strong enough for such a journey. Here I was in hospital, diverted from the suicide road onto a bypass that might keep me alive for a little while, but I knew this was not the end of it. I knew I would try and get there again.

A doctor came in and started poking around in my cuts. It hurt but I didn't care, I wanted it to. This whole experience hurt and that was exactly how it should be. He had shinny metal tools that looked like tweezers and he was pulling bits of severed flesh about. He mumbled something and left me there, bleeding on the white sheet that I was laying on. After a long time he came back with another doctor and they both had another poke and another look and then they finally spoke to me.

"We're going to need the plastics surgeon to come out and sew you up, you've severed arteries." So that was why they were bleeding more than any other cut. I guess I knew I'd done something like that, I guess I had done it on purpose. It seemed to be that the plastics surgeon was not on duty but they had to call him in to sort me out. I imagined that he might be in bed, that he was sleeping and now he had to be disturbed because of me. I felt guilty, yet I also felt important. Now I wasn't the only one that knew of my pain, now all these doctors and nurses knew. …But I felt equally alone.

Hours later another doctor came in through the curtains and went to work straight away. He pulled at the inside of my arm and once he had what he needed in between his tongs he stitched bits of it up. I don't remember them giving me any injections to take the pain away yet I coped with the pain, it just didn't matter. The pain was constant and what the doctor was doing didn't really make any difference. I didn't care that he had to sew up my arteries. I didn't care that I was going to have scars. This was what Steve did; this was running its natural course.

Stitched up, I thought that I would be free to go, but they made me sit in a waiting room so that they could get a psychiatrist to speak to me. I agreed to wait. I guess I wanted help. I guess I was ready to try anything, just please make the urge to die go away, make my skin look better, make my life less lonely. …But how a psychiatrist was going to do all that I didn't know. I wondered if they would want to keep me in hospital. I wondered if I wanted that. Perhaps I should have been locked up. Perhaps it would be best for my continued safety. Perhaps I had to be stopped from doing this again, locked in a padded cell where I could not harm myself anymore, but I knew that was all a little far fetched. They didn't just lock people up anymore. This was the year 2001 after all.

I waited hours before I was seen. I should have been tired as it was the early hours of the morning by now but I didn't feel anything as definable as fatigue. My mind was working through my whole life, thinking about how bad things were, thinking about what I might have to tell the shrink when he finally arrived. I felt that a mind was all I was, that I had no body just a sinking soul. I looked down at my bandaged arms and could hardly believe that they were attached to me. If only. If only I had escaped this body, this ugly face. If only I had died.

"Stephen?"

A man came in to the waiting room and I looked up to see him. He wore a brown suit jacket and brown cords. He looked to be about thirty-five, quite young I thought. He was slim but his face seemed to have retained some puppy fat. He wore glasses. I was glad for his sympathetic air; his voice and words were kind. I needed sympathy; I needed to be treated with care. Wrap me up in cotton wool and leave me there. Let me make a chrysalis and stay there for years while my face mends, while my mind forgets. Let me emerge beautiful and healed.

131

"Yes." My voice was weak and when the words came it shocked me that I could still talk.

"Is it ok if we have a little chat?"

"Yes." I nodded.

I was glad that they had taken me seriously, that they were going to help me now, that I would be cared for. I was glad that these doctors never slept.

He talked to me for at least an hour asking what would soon become very hackneyed questions. Did you really want to die? What happened that made you do it? Have you tried it before? Do you hear voices? I answered them all truthfully; I didn't hold back. I told him that I wanted to die, that this was not just a cry for help, that I really thought I had the courage I had been waiting on to finally slit my wrists, to finally get out of this horrible life. I told him that I had a wife but was divorced and that we had split up six months ago. I told him that I didn't think that was the reason. I didn't know the reason, yet I told him about my face, about how my skin made me a prisoner. I told him that I had tried it before. I told him that I didn't hear voices.

"Do you think you might try it again?"

"Not now, not yet." I meant that, I couldn't bear to do it again. Suicidal thoughts are like a journey up a mountain. You know when it is coming, you know you're making your way up, you can feel it all brewing you can spot the danger signs. Looking down you see your life getting further and further out of reach, and you just keep going up and up until you reach its peak where there is nothing left, but to act upon it. That peak is the scariest place, high on despair you look down and you get vertigo and there is only one way down. You're going to fall and fall hard, you are going to have to die. I was over the peak now, I was on my way down the other side, and I had survived a moment that would not yet come again.

"I'm going to refer you to the Letchworth mental health team and they will give you help and support. I'll try and get you an appointment as soon as possible. You are not on any medication are you?"

"No."

"Then I'm going to prescribe for you Paroxetine, it's an antidepressant. I hope that will help you."

He wrote a prescription out and handed it to me. I took it with shaking fingers.

"Ok. Remember if you ever feel like doing something like this again please just come to A and E and you can see the duty psychiatrist at any time. Ok. Well good luck Stephen please take care of yourself."

...And that was it. That was the experience over with. Now I was, once again, tossed back into the world like an over small fish on a fly-fishing trip. I wasn't bad enough to stay in hospital, I was not a risk to myself or anyone else at that very moment and so I was given back to my life, to try again to live.

I left the room and made my way out through the emergency department, past bleeding fingers and fragile swollen limbs, out through the double doors to the outside world. It was light outside. I had been in the hospital all night. I had not slept and now my head was fuzzy. My feet dragged as I walked, but where was I walking to? I had no money and nowhere to go but home, which was about five miles away. I hadn't planned this part, I never did. I had to get someone to take me home and I decided that it should be my sister. I could tell her what I had done, but I wasn't going to tell anyone else. No one would benefit from that little piece of tragic information. I wasn't doing this to hurt people and I remembered all too well the damage that a suicide attempt caused. I didn't want to worry my parents, my grandmother, not even my sister, but I needed her help now, and I needed, for all the selfish reasons, to unload this horrible little event on someone else's shoulders.

"Jane, I need a favour. Could you pick me up from the hospital?" Silence for a painful moment and then she said:

"Yes of course, but I'll have to take the kids to school first.'

My nieces, of which there were three by this time, would never know what their uncle Steve had done. They would never know there was anything wrong with me. Depression is practically invisible.

"What have you done?" The question finally arose.

"I cut my arms. Don't tell mum."

She agreed to pick me up at about nine o'clock and I said I would wait at the main entrance doors. I had no idea that it was only seven o'clock until I saw the clock behind the reception desk. This was turning out to be a long ordeal and wasn't one I wanted to repeat, but I didn't want this existence either. I didn't want to have to explain to work why I was not in. I did not want to be answerable to so many people. I didn't want to go back to my lonely house, alone, alone with so many troubled thoughts, but that was the only life on offer. I did not feel reborn I felt regurgitated, a waste product of a person forced to live his putrid life despite every attempt to leave. ...But I was getting help now wasn't I? Apparently.

134

I got the pills from the pharmacy and sat waiting for my lift feeling exposed, feeling paranoid. Did everyone know what I had done? Were they all looking at the ugly skinned guy with the slashed wrists? I tried to hide, making my body smaller, hunched up and tight trying not to watch everyone that went past. I decided to read through the information sheet that was with my medication. It was interesting reading.

Seroxat, Paroxetine: A selective serotonin reuptake inhibitor. Side effects include nausea, somnolence, sweating, tremor, asthenia, dizziness, dry mouth, insomnia and male sexual dysfunction. It all sounded quite awful, but I knew that it has to list everything no matter how unlikely the side effects were. Every drug could cause side effects. Reading further, however, I was shocked to see that other side effects include nervousness, panic attacks, and suicidal tendencies! Great, so the drugs might make me better, they might make me worse, I looked forward to finding out what they would do for me with much pessimism.

My sister spoke to me kindly but didn't ask me any questions, and I didn't want to talk about it. We glossed over what had actually happened and spoke as if things were still fine. They were far from fine however, this was the beginning of my misery years, not that I had ever really been happy.

My sister asked me if I would like to come back to hers' rather than go home to an empty house, and I said I would. I didn't want to be alone, I wanted to be looked after, but she warned me, my mother would be there. She was there correcting her book on my sister's computer. I had to think deeply, was I going to tell her and if not, what excuse could I give for being off work and needing my sister to pick me up? I think it became pretty clear that I would not be able to keep it from her. I began to see my sister's anguish as well. It wasn't fair to have burdened her with this secret.

When I walked into my sister's living room with bandages on my arms my mother turned from the computer screen with a look of puzzled horror.

"You've been cutting yourself again?"

"It's a little worse than that."

My mother seemed cross.   I never could judge her reactions.

"You've tried to kill yourself?"

And at last I found my tears.

The Red Herring.

My house was such a quiet place that I could hear my own breathing above all else. The gentle electrical hum of the refrigerator the only noise that proved the house was still switched on. I sat on my sofa looking out of my window, feeling that everything outside that window was far more distant than a mere opening of a latch. I saw the birds flying in and out of the bushes completely silently, no wings flapping nor leafs parting. I watched the wind making the hedges slowly dance, but it was not accompanied by sound. No wonder the world felt so distant from me.

I knew there was a world out there somewhere, people having lives - people doing things. I racked my brains to work out what made them so different. What were they doing right that I was doing wrong? How do people use up their time? ...So many hours - lying in bed - wandering my rooms - waiting.

It seemed that I was waiting for something to happen. Perhaps for them it had already happened. Perhaps, somewhere out there, things were happening all the time, but my life was going nowhere. Perhaps I would have to do something to make it happen? ...But the world seemed so very far away...

I used to be content to watch movies, but I hadn't watched anything in months. I no longer enjoyed anything. All I did was write short prose, and when I wasn't writing I was drinking, listening to music and staring out of whichever window I was closest to. Life wasn't like the movies. A day on Earth lasts twenty-four hours, a day in the movies mere minutes. I am no actor. Life was just this; secular, boring, lonely and miserable. Real life lasts for years.

I didn't want to be alone anymore; it had lost all of its former grace. I had finished my novel, it was not accepted, I had surfed the internet and listened to my music, but there is only so much I can take of my own company. Loneliness, it would appear, is my one great weakness. I need my space, that much I already knew, but this wasn't 'space' this was expulsion. Being on my own would have been fine so long as I had someone to tell about it, but my mother had become the only company I ever got. Plus, she had a great way of annoying me. Your mother should not be your only friend.

My sister would invite me over quite regularly on a Sunday for dinner - sometimes I accepted other times I just didn't want to leave the house. I wore make up every day at work but so long as I wasn't seeing anyone for the whole weekend, I figured that I could give my skin a rest. I would clean my face and put Savlon over it, sometimes putting on so much that it no longer sank in and left my face white with cream. Then I would write short prose on my computer or surf the net trying not to think about it.

Sometimes there would be a knock at the door and I would go into panic mode. I would jump up, turn off the stereo, and run quietly up the stairs and into my bedroom. I would stay there and wait, as silently as I could be, for whoever it was to go. Sometimes they wouldn't go. I would be behind my bedroom door, trying not to breathe, my heart racing. I would tip toe across the landing and into the bathroom, having a quick look at myself in the mirror to see if I could be seen but then realising that it was just not possible.

"Steve?" My name called through the letterbox. They knew I was in because I had nowhere to go. Well, I could be at the supermarket, was I not allowed to have a life?

"Steve?" I would know who it was by now, but it would make no difference. It could be Michael driving over on the off chance that I would be in. It could be my sister's husband inviting me for dinner, there to pick me up and take me to their house. It could be my mother just trying to give me some company so that I wasn't alone all the time. Didn't they realise that I hated uninvited visits? I never answered unless I had been given about an hour's notice. There was no way I would answer to a cold call.

Then the phone would ring. Did they think I was stupid? There was no way I was going to answer the phone and give them proof I was in the house. It was them calling me on their mobile, it was obvious and I was not falling for it. I would let it ring and ring and finally they would give up. Shit! What if they went into the garden they would see the computer on through the window?

I would creep down the stairs craning my neck to see through the living room window before they saw me. If there was no one in the garden I could quickly get to the computer, turn off the monitor and race back up the stairs.

I would listen for the sound of their car to start up and drive away, but I would not rest. I would not go downstairs for a good hour just in case they were still there waiting for me to come back. I would stay in the bedroom lying on my bed wishing my life wasn't like this. I wished that I could see people, that I could go out, but I just couldn't. I didn't want to go through the make up routine every single day of my life and it was only at the weekends that I could leave it off.

I never answered the phone anymore. I didn't want to talk to anyone. I didn't want to know what was going on with my family and I certainly didn't want to know what was going on in the world at large. When I did speak to them they told me off for ignoring their calls, and then they would talk, reminding me of why I usually didn't answer. I wanted to be left alone. I just wanted to hide away and write.

'I seclude myself in my own loneliness, shutting myself off from any chance. Stay inside - it's safer on your own. Keep myself in misery. It's the only me I've ever known....'

Sometimes the solitude would get too much for me and I would put a little make up on, just enough to be seen by strangers (I preferred to look ugly in front of strangers than in front of family, friends or work colleagues) and then I could brave the world and go to the supermarket. I went to the supermarket quite a lot. Some times going to Sainsburys was my Friday or Saturday night on the town. I would go there after work or later that night and would always buy alcohol. Ice cream and alcohol were the only essentials I needed. Of course I would buy other stuff, I was eating a few stable meals a week, but having to get the shopping on my bike or on foot meant I couldn't get much, and cider was heavy.

I was drinking a lot because why not? I went to work, I had the money and I had no one to stop me. The only pleasure I had was to drink and to sing a long with the Smiths, the only way to make misery more acceptable.

I was still thinking about suicide. Everyday for at least half of the time my thoughts were focused on ending my life. It was hard to live with, but I was coping. Although I still hated my life, I hadn't reached that peak again. There were little mountains with smaller peaks and at the top of those I would go to the bathroom and slash my arms. It seemed that I was doing it now for the smallest of reasons. I was doing it at least once a week. Sitting on the toilet seat, lashing out at myself, taking all my self-hatred and all my misery and making it physical. I liked that it was leaving me with scars; I liked the two biggest scars that severing my arteries had caused. They were like tattoos, like war wounds. I didn't want anyone else to see them but I liked to look at them, I deserved them, every one.

I was still waiting for an appointment with a psychologist but I had a social worker called Owen that came to see me at home once a week. I could tell him anything and I did. I told him things I had never told anyone and although he could not really help he was at least an ear to chew off. I told him about my skin, one of my deepest secrets, and he listened and he said that they might be able to help me. At least having a social worker meant that they were keeping and eye on me. They knew that I was serious when I tried to end my life. They knew I was seriously depressed.

Were the new pills working? I wasn't sure. I wasn't sure if hating my own face was a product of depression or whether I was depressed because of my face. I could not separate the two. If my skin were better would I be suddenly cured of depression? I didn't know, though I didn't really believe that I would, for it would not suddenly fill me with a passion for life. I was depressed because I was trapped on this world and the fact that I was trapped in this skin just made it all worse. Perhaps the medication was working; perhaps it was taking the suicidal urges away? I hadn't tried to kill myself again despite the fact that nothing in my life had changed and, if anything, things were worse. I was writing regularly, I was eating and sleeping ok, but my skin was really getting me down. The time I was spending in the bathroom each day was getting ridiculous. I had to get up two hours early for work just so that I had time to sort it out and spent just as long on it each night. It was always on my mind and my mind was full of darkness.

I got an appointment to see a psychologist and I had every intention of going, but I was having a bad day. I tried to get ready to go but I kept thinking about it, thinking of all the things I would have to say and I started to panic. I looked awful. I couldn't make my face go right and the time was ticking. It was time I should be there and there I was sitting on my bathroom floor with a shaving mirror in front of my face, on the verge of tears. There were so many areas of my skin that I had picked and squeezed and poked that I had ended up with wounds that couldn't be covered up. It was no use. I felt physically sick; my heart was racing so fast I could hardly breathe. As soon as I decided that I wouldn't go, the better I felt. I went downstairs and rang the mental health unit.

"Hi, I had an appointment for two o'clock but I can't make it; I can't leave the house."

"Well don't you think you should have told us earlier? Now that's a wasted appointment that someone else could have had." The lady on the end of the phone sounded quite annoyed. I couldn't believe that they would be like that; I thought they would understand. It really shocked me and it made me feel worse. If they were going to be like that I didn't want their help.

That same day I went to the doctors. I decided to do something once and for all. I would tell him how spots were ruining my life, but how could I tell him the complete truth. How could I explain that my skin was actually too thin and you could see through it? How could I tell him about the redness and the swelling? I would keep it simple and just ask for something for the spots.

As I told the doctor about it I started to cry. He said that he didn't really think I had any real problem with spots. He said everyone gets a few spots from time to time and I tried to explain how they ruined my life. I broke into tears, crying pitifully. I couldn't hold it in any longer, all those hours of staring into mirrors; I just couldn't take it anymore. I buried my face in my hands and I wished I could stay that way, I wished I didn't ever have to ever be seen.

He gave me some acne cream and I figured I could use it as well as everything else I put on my face. I was thankful for it yet I knew it wouldn't help. I guess somehow I knew, despite what my eyes and brain told me, that there was really nothing wrong with my skin.

That didn't help me to feel any less depressed. I was in almost constant solitude. Loneliness was a big issue. I was hiding from life and had no life to speak of. I would go to work and come home alone, it was just me, and I was depressing company.

In a sudden revelation I thought of internet dating. I hadn't thought of it before and I don't know why I suddenly thought of it now, but that didn't matter. I was sure it was the answer and so I started to search for sites. 'Dating', 'personals', whatever searches I could think of, following links and adverts and soon finding out that there were loads of these sites around. I actually started to get excited and excitement was something I had not felt in years. I truly believed that this would be the way I would find the elusive 'one'.

Most of the dating sites asked you to create a profile before you could search them. I would fill in the criteria, male looking for female, aged twenty to thirty in Hertfordshire and click the button and... 'Create your profile for free to begin searching hundreds of personals!' Well, what the hell, I would set up a profile and I would start to look and she would be there, the 'one' would be there I was certain of it. So I bought myself a web cam and took shots of myself trying to look good. My skin looked perfect in the web cam pictures and I was quite pleased with them. So I downloaded them onto the site and filled in the online form. It asked for your basic details, your age, height and job. I didn't lie although I started to feel that I might not be what most of these girls would be looking for. Then it came to filling in an empty box with whatever you wanted to say about yourself. This was the hard bit. How could I make myself seem interesting? How could I make myself sound like less of a freak? 'Young depressive with social phobia wishes to not meet anyone because he's too damn ugly anyway.' I thought about it for ages, pacing around the house. I wrote things out on paper and changed them and rewrote them and, eventually, I had it...

'Hi, my name is Steve, I'm looking for someone that I can share things with, having a drink and putting the world to wrongs. I'm very much into alternative music and like to go and see bands live. I also like to write and have finished one novel and lots of short prose. I'm not a 'laddish' kind of guy, which hopefully is a good thing. If you are similar then please get in touch.'

It was simple, informative, and slightly humorous. I was pleased. The best thing was, however, that now I had done that I could search the site to see if there were any girls on there that would suit me. I was the most optimistic I had been in a long time. I was doing something about my life. I was giving myself a chance to actually have a life. I wasn't listening to the Stephen that wanted me dead, I was Mr. Optimistic today and I was looking for my other half.

The good thing about online dating, I thought, was that you could be selective. You can look for someone that is exactly what you are looking for and if they don't fit your profile of a perfect partner you can choose not to get involved without hurting anyone's feelings. It seemed perfect, but what it also makes you is very choosy. I ploughed through the profiles and none of them seemed like my kind of person, or if they did, there was a photograph of them that I just wasn't attracted to. They might sound nice but did they like alternative music? They might like alternative music but were they pretty? They might be pretty but have they ever read a book? Was that book anything that I might like? It was hopeless. I spent literally hours looking through page after page and saw no one that fitted my criteria. I came down to Earth with a bump. Misery came back to slap any ideas of happiness away. I was too damned ill to have a girlfriend anyway, and having no one, being so lonely made me feel so damned ill. What was I thinking of looking for a girl? I had nothing to offer anyone. I couldn't even drive to go see them. I couldn't have sex, not just with my history but the pills I was on were having some strange effects. I was pathetic.

Feeling that I had nothing to offer the world killed my survival instinct, if ever I had one. Why live when you were as ugly and as useless as me? My job was unskilled, my family all wished I was different, I was a failure in love, and I was sexually rejected. Not that Carey ever left me alone to live my so-called life. She would phone me, suddenly out of the blue she would call and she would tell me that she had started cutting herself again and that Jude didn't understand her. What did she want me to do about it? She would talk for hours and as I had little else, I would listen and I would try to help, but really I couldn't and shouldn't have anything to do with her problems.

She asked me if she could come over one day and I was dreading that she wanted to take more stuff. She said she just wanted to talk. Jude drove her to my house and she had asked him to pick her up in three hours. I wondered what he thought of this, I wondered what anyone would think of this. My family would all disapprove, they all told me that I should tell Carey to leave me alone and that I shouldn't even speak to her anymore. ...But here she was, for three hours, pouring out her heart.

She was dreadfully unhappy and all I could do to help was to empathize. I told her about my failed attempt at my life and she asked if it was her fault. I said it wasn't. She had been cutting her arms and Jude had hidden all the knives. I wondered if we were both complete loonies.

"Do you miss me?" She asked. I had to look at her to see if she was being

sincere. It was just like her to say something like that to make me look a fool. If I had said that I did she would probably laugh at me. I had to think about the answer for every reason. I didn't know if I missed her or not.

"I miss someone," I said.

"Oh thanks."

"Well what do you expect me to say? We got divorced. Anyway it's all right for you, you went with Jude straight away."

"Mmm. Have yourself a girlfriend yet?"

"No."

"Why not, you're a bit slow aren't you?"

"How would I meet anyone? I never go out."

"You should go out."

"Well, I don't, I can't go anywhere on my own can I?"

"You have the internet don't you?"

I wasn't going to get into that conversation. In fact, discussing my love life or lack of it, with my ex-wife just didn't appeal to me, but she seemed to love talking about hers. She told me how Jude wanted to see his kid but his ex wasn't allowing him access. She told me how his ex was getting nasty and threatening all sorts of things. I wished that I didn't care but I did still have an ounce of feeling for her. I wanted her to be happy, but one thing I really wanted to know I would never ask her. I wanted to know if they were sleeping together. I wanted to know if she had finally lost her virginity and to him not me. If so, and I imagined it was, what had been so wrong with me?

She left and left me with all sorts of troubled feelings. I cut my arms with my faithful Stanley blade, slowly so I felt the pain, watching it dent and then pierce my skin, dragging it over my wrist to a trail of blood. I was doing that a lot lately; every little thing sparked me off. I didn't even try to stop myself anymore, I just did it and I always wore long sleeves despite the onset of summer.

I was feeling close to the edge but someone had a hold of me, something was stopping me from jumping, or were they getting ready to push?

One night I got home from work, threw my bag on the floor, got the cider from the fridge and sat straight down to my computer. I drank and I checked my e-mails.

'You have a message at Dating Partners.com'

Oh my God! I couldn't believe it, it had been ages since I put myself on there and despite looking most nights I had not seen any likely candidates. I realised that meant something though. I probably wouldn't be interested in this person and more importantly this person wouldn't really be interested in me. They were mistaken. They didn't realise what I was, they didn't realise I was such a loser.

I followed the link and it went to the site but I had to pay if I wanted to read the message. So that's how they make their money! There was a cheap three-day trial option and that seemed like the best course of action, but first I wanted to look at her profile to see if I had any idea why she would contact me. I got her profile up, and straight away realised that I had not seen this girl on there before. She was from London. I never searched for people from London, but that was fine; I could travel on the train to see her. There I was jumping the gun; I'm surprised that I hadn't already got us married with kids.

Her name was Andie, she was twenty-five. Her picture wasn't very clear but she was smiling in it and she had long blonde hair. I read the profile and it said she wanted someone to give her a ride on a Vespa; well I couldn't help her there. It also said that she liked music like the Smiths and Morrissey. I certainly wanted to read her message. There was definitely a chance this could work.

I paid to read what she had to say. I typed in my credit card number and I clicked on my message box...

'Hey! I liked your profile! I live in London but I'm originally from South Carolina in the states. I've been here for two years and work for a University. I am really into 80's music like the Smiths, Depeche Mode and New Order and I go to a lot of gigs here in London. What are you in to? If you're still looking for someone I would really like to hear from you. Andie.'

I was frozen. I sat staring at the computer screen unsure what to do. I was excited but I was also afraid. This had come at a bad time - I wasn't well. I didn't know if I could socialise with anyone right now, especially a stranger. If we arranged a date I would probably panic about my face so much that I wouldn't be able to leave the house. If I got as far as reaching the pub, or wherever we arranged to

148

meet, I would probably sit there like I was now, dumbstruck with nothing to say. Yet this was what I had been waiting for wasn't it? Did I not put myself on the site with a belief that I would meet my soul mate? This could be her and here I was sitting, paralysed, unsure whether I should answer.

I got up from the computer and put some heavy music on, something that would be louder than my thoughts. Perhaps I would get my answer if it were strong enough to yell over the din. I drank cider from a glass that I was topping up after every other gulp. I paced my living room and I looked in the mirror standing on my sofa, staring into it and posing in different faces. Could I let anyone see this face? Was it as bad as I made out? No one else seemed to notice, or they were too polite to say. My mother never understood when I said I had bad skin. Maybe I did a good job on the make up.

I ran upstairs to my bedroom and looked in the mirror there. Was this a more accurate reflection? I looked a little worse in this one. I hadn't removed my make up yet but I always liked to do that early in the evening to give my skin the longest possible time to heal. Of course that meant that I had to pretend I was out if anyone came to the house. I went into the bathroom and washed my face without turning on the light. It was still light outside but in the bathroom it was quite dull. Would this girl be disappointed if she saw me in the flesh? I didn't look so bad in this light.

I went into the bedroom, took up my notepad that was by the bed, and flicked through the pages. I wrote ideas for stories in there; sometimes I would write them out before typing them up. Sometimes I would have such a vivid dream that I would wake up with it still affecting my mind and I wrote it down in that book. I remember one about a science lab where they were keeping zombies. It was a white, clean, sterile place yet there were these vile disgusting creatures that were barely human, putrid, rotting in dirty, ripped up clothes. ...And there were naked girls strapped to beds.

149

Then the zombies were let out and they went straight to the girls and they viciously raped them. I woke up in a panic, sweating and gasping. I hated that my mind had thought up such a horrible vision. I wondered what it said about my mental health. It stayed with me all day and I thought of making it into a story, but that wasn't my style. The only horror stories I had written were the vampire tales I wrote in my early years. I didn't want to dwell on things like that. Nowadays my stories were more like parables.

There was one interesting thing that had come from my dreams. I had reoccurring dreams about people finding the bodies that I had buried. I never dreamt about actually killing anyone but I dreamt of the police or searchers finding the black bin bags that contained the body parts. I dreamt of a dog pulling an arm up from the ground, but most important was the fear that I felt to have been found out. It was so real. I awoke actually feeling guilty, actually really worried that it had been true and that they really had found evidence against me. I had to try and rationalise it to myself "Steve, you have not killed anyone," but sometimes the emotion was with me all day. Sometimes I just had that sinking feeling in my gut. This got me thinking and a new novel was growing inside my head. I had started to plan a scenario that could grow into a real story. Perhaps my next book would be the one to get me noticed.

I lay on the bed and started to write possible replies to the girl that had sent me a message. It wouldn't be fair to her to not reply. Yet it would not be fair to subject her to me either. Perhaps I should send an apologetic answer explaining how she should not really waste her time with me. Yes that's what I would do. I would protect myself and protect her.

I wrote reply after reply and finally I was happy with one. It was a friendly message that said thank you for writing to me, we have similar music tastes, but I must warn you that I suffer with depression. It said other things about

150

my favourite films and such. It was keeping my options open - not sounding too keen, but sounding interesting, yet warning her of the one thing I could not change. I had told her straight up and time would tell whether this scared her off or not. It didn't.

She wrote me an e-mail back saying thank you for being so honest and that she also suffers with depression, and guess what? We have something in common because we are both on the same meds! Oh joy. What fun we could have! ...But I really believed, at the time, that this could be a good thing. I wanted a girl that was different to most of those ads, those girls that said, "I want someone to make me laugh, someone that doesn't take life too seriously." Well if you can't take life seriously what the hell can you be serious about? Life is serious; life is the only thing we have. I don't want to be a comedian; I want to have deep meaningful conversations about life, death, music and films. I don't only want someone that I can be happy with, but someone that I can be miserable with as well. Andie... are you the one?

I wrote back then she wrote back and through the next week we ended up finding out a lot about each other over e-mails. She said how she looks forward to going to work because she gets to read my messages. Nothing I was saying was putting her off me, but of course, I didn't tell her everything. So we had an e-mail frenzy for a week until she finally asked me out on a date. The Cure were playing that weekend in Hyde Park, did I want to go? Yes I wanted to go! I wanted to meet her, I wanted to see the Cure, and she said she had tickets booked. I was excited again.

The day before the show and I get an e-mail saying that she's not sure she can meet me, and so I e-mail her back saying that I was nervous too but that we should definitely go, that it would be a great day. I convinced her. I wish I hadn't. I should have sensed that she was bad news.

151

So came the day of the date and I got up extra early so that I could sort out my face and get out of the house. I was terribly worried that I might have one of my bad days but despite utter panic my make up went on quite well and hid all the blemishes I could find. I wasn't going to settle though. I kept walking from room to room holding the shaving mirror, checking myself out in the different rooms as each one had a different light. When I realised that I did not look like a freak I calmed down a little, though only a little. I was nervous as hell but that was to be expected. I felt incompetent and naive. I felt vulnerable, on show to a disapproving world, and I was trying to have a life despite a disapproving 'other me' that told me I was just putting off the inevitable pain.

I caught the train, I wandered through Oxford Street looking for this little pub we had planned to meet in, and to my surprise I found it easily. It was quite dark in the pub, which made me feel a little more comfortable, but I was early. I got myself a beer and sat down on a stall that faced the door. I noticed my hands were shaking and my insides were doing the flips. I kept staring round the pub looking to see if she was already there and I hadn't seen her. I realised that I wouldn't recognise her if she were. I sent her a text message:

I am here already. Are you ok?

She answered:

Yes - I'm here too - I'm looking right at you!

My gut did a summersault and I started to look around the pub trying not to look as if I was stupid. There were some blonde girls in there but none were on their own and none seemed to be looking at me. My phone signalled another text:

Not really! I'm on my way - be 5 minutes.

I had been fooled! I saw the funny side of it but it didn't help my nerves. Now I was really anxious knowing that I would see her walk through the door any second. Was this her? A girl dressed all in black with a large leather belt and blonde hair, smiling at me, coming towards me.

"Steve?"

"Yes! Hi- Andie. You look lovely." I blurted out, saying exactly what I thought when I saw her without filtering the words. Then I decided it was ok to have said that, it was just a compliment. I couldn't remember how to do this dating thing, I felt like a fish out of water. I felt like a nervous little boy. She was two years younger than me yet she seemed so much more grown up; she'd probably had so much more experience in such situations. I felt like I was looking up to her already. She was too good for me; I fumbled with my words and spilt some of my beer as I put it down on a table for two.

"So how are you?" She asked with a soft American accent. I liked her voice and I thought she was very pretty. We talked quite easily together too. I lost some of my nerves as I felt words drifting out from my mouth and saw her smiling back at me and laughing as if I were witty. We talked about music, films and 'Big Brother' and how we both liked to watch people and try to work them out. Then we came to the inevitable - talking about how we had been affected by depression. It felt good to be able to tell someone though she was given the filtered down version. I didn't tell her that I had tried to kill myself, just that I was depressed, on the same medication that she was and that I cut myself sometimes. She told me the same. We had both had the same experience and this was the first time I had spoken about my depression and seen understanding in someone's eyes. I thought that we understood each other completely. We spoke about it for a while but did not dwell. It needed to be said and it needed to be put aside, then it was done with.

It was a very warm and sunny day and we walked to Hyde Park holding hands and chatting on the way. I felt confident about the date, it seemed to be going fine and she seemed to like me. I certainly liked her and we were going to see the Cure! It seemed to be so perfect and that's how it was set up in my mind now. Despite my nerves, despite the hard time I had getting ready, despite my lack of dating experience I really thought that this was all so wonderful.

In the queue to get in I stood behind her and put my arms round her waist. She turned her head around and we kissed. So she did like me. This really was the start of something. I wasn't so mistaken. Not yet.

Seeing the Cure live would have been great with whoever I was with but with the prospect of having a relationship with this girl, it just made it all the better. Quite frankly, and quite stupidly, I had fallen for her instantly. I put all my eggs in this one basket because I had no other baskets to consider. I hated being alone; I hated how I felt about myself, and here was Andie, a free spirited American girl that liked me, that wanted to spend time with me. That danced with me to 'Just Like Heaven' in the hot evening dusk. Well I was hers already.

Love - formed on looks and voices and desperation to be loved is not a great foundation. Add to that a lack of self worth and a penchant for depression, and you have yourself a lethal cocktail. I didn't see any of this at the time. I thought that I had just been very, very lucky, and quite right when I said and believed that I would find 'the one' on the internet. I decided that this was her. She had no say in the matter.

At the end of the show we both walked out of the park together, both on a massive high (something I hadn't felt for years) and Andie took me by my hands and held me and said, "Come home with me."

That shook my anxiety into a panic. I wanted this relationship to progress but if she wanted me to have sex with her it could spoil everything. It would wash the mask away, and quite literally too; I had no make up with me, but this was my chance wasn't it? My chance to be loved and I was so starved of affection. I didn't want this night, this day to end. I wanted to go with her, but could I, could Steve do this? I felt a sudden bout of confidence, and as the words got close to my lips I changed them to accommodate my fear.

"Just to hold each other." I said.

"Ok." She answered and I believed her. I believed myself that it would be just like that. That we could hold each other, talk and sleep and not wake up alone.

We took a taxi and we arrived at the block of flats where she lived. She led me up the stairs, still holding hands and we went in. Her room was quite big and very untidy, there were clothes and CDs littered around. There were music posters on the walls that were not put up straight and were falling down. Andie was the first in and started picking up some of the stuff and chucking it in a corner. She turned on the big stand-alone fan that was really needed as the warm day had heated the room up uncomfortably.

"Choose some CDs from the pile, I'll be back in a minute", and so I was there, in this stranger's home looking through a CD collection that looked very much like my own. I choose four CDs and put them by the stereo. Then I sat on her bed.

When Andie came back she was wearing a red silk robe. I guess I knew that something was going to happen, that my plea to 'just hold each other' was not going to be respected, and can a guy ever say no to sex? A woman is not thought of badly if they say no but what would Andie say if I refused to go down that road. She would be offended; she would wonder what was so wrong with her. She would think that I was a freak, but if we did do that then she would perhaps find out something else bad about me - I didn't know how to make love. I didn't know if I was physically or mentally able to do it.

She put on a CD and then she got onto the bed prowling up to me and starting to kiss my neck and then my lips. She started to remove my clothes. It was happening. At twenty-seven, with a girl I had only met that day; I was going to lose my sacred virginity. It was strange, surreal. I didn't believe that it was actually happening, that I was actually in my body. I found the whole experience quite unnerving and my mind wandered. I thought about things I didn't want to think about - animals shagging in some nature documentary, clips of a porno film I had been subjected to at a teenage party. I didn't want this, not really, and so I stopped and we just kissed and held each other. Before long Andie was asleep and I was lying there wondering what she would think of me now. I wondered if this would ever happen again and whether I wanted it to. ...But I truly believed that I loved this girl already and we had just had a wonderful day together. I allowed myself a smile and as I listened to the hum of the fan, I looked out of the window into the black night sky over London and I thought, this is a new dimension. Steve's life had just changed.

I was on a high the next day and after lying in bed with Andie chatting about what we would do if we won the lottery; I left so that I didn't miss my mother's birthday meal. It was a scorching hot day and although I felt good I was on the tube train flushed and sweating and worrying about what I looked like. I really wanted to get home now and get in front of a mirror. I needed to wash the make up off and start again. I tried to make myself smaller and less conspicuous but there were eyes burning me, coming from everywhere. I hate tube trains at the best of times but in that heat and with yesterday's clothes on, I felt terribly claustrophobic.

I texted Andie when I got home, telling her what a wonderful day I had and saying that I couldn't wait to see her again. She replied with similar enthusiasm. I'm sure the pain and worry had been completely lifted from my eyes, because my mother could tell how well the date went without having to ask. She did ask however and I grinned back.

Suicide was still on my mind but it seemed ridiculous to actually act on it. I had something to live for now didn't I? I seldom had anything to live for, anything that made the pain of life go away, but here was a chance and I was going to take it. I went to work all day and somehow I got through the day without thinking of killing myself. Why kill myself when I had the chance to be with Andie? It would not make sense to end my life when there were good things happening, things I enjoyed. I didn't enjoy much but I did enjoy being with her. I wanted to see what would happen next.

We kept in touch by text and I had my phone with me at work. It made the day go by so much happier. Then she e-mailed me to ask me on another date, to see Peter Murphy with her in London, at the same venue that I had seen Tori Amos. I guessed she must like me, she wasn't put off by my lack of experience, and she wanted to be my girlfriend. Well that's what I thought.

I know I was stupidly blind to the dangers. I know that I completely let my guard down, but I wanted it so badly. I was lonely and depressed and here was a girl, a lonely and depressed girl and together we could be great. Didn't I ever think that two people with such dark minds together could be

157

dangerous? I did, but I wanted the danger. Give us a few weeks together and then we could do it. Here was a girl that I could make the pact with.

In my book 'Personal Demons' I had a scene where the lead character tries to convince his girlfriend to make a suicide pact with him. He wanted to die with someone, rather than die alone. I could see that happening with Andie and I and I wanted it. I was looking for an excuse to kill myself again. I always look for excuses, for reasons that would make it easier on my family when they ask the inevitable question... 'Why?' Let them blame my death on Andie if it made it better for them, it couldn't hurt her if she was dead too.

I met Andie in a pub close to the venue and she hugged me and said that I looked great. I was wearing blue low rise flared jeans and a black shirt. I had a lot of make up on. We sat and talked and kissed and then we went on to the show. I loved that venue. Despite how I feel about organised religion I do like churches, they are, in fact, quite beautiful. I led Andie along, holding her hand as she walked behind me and we sat down, close together on the pews.

The music filled the building, reflecting off the stone walls, reaching out to the high ceiling. There were Gothic sounds and Peter Murphy's ethereal voice calling out to the audience's souls. "I am convinced Peter Murphy is a vampire," Andie said, and I smiled back.

"If there is such things as vampires, then he is one."

It was only a few songs into the set that Andie took my hand and pulled me up. She wanted to go. She seemed quite distressed.

I didn't understand what the matter was but when we got out of the main room and into the hallway she began to calm down.

"I just couldn't sit there anymore with all those people." She explained and I said it was ok and that I understood. She had suffered the start of a panic attack and I knew what they felt like - I had them nearly every morning.

We spent the rest of the show in the hallway drinking beer. At least I was drinking beer, I don't remember if Andie was. I don't remember much more actually. I remember being back at her flat and I remember feeling very pissed. I think she was as well and she had a bottle of wine, which we drank too. I picked out a Tori Amos CD and asked her to put it on saying that if I could lie in bed with her and listen to that then, I might just have a little slice of happiness. …And with the sound of Tori's piano and heartfelt voice we lay in each other's arms and I said the most stupid thing I could have said. I said:

"I love you."

Perhaps it was the beer talking. Perhaps I was taken in by the fact that she was from a different country and had a different life style. Perhaps I liked the dizzy heights of London. Perhaps I just associated Andie with two very good music concerts and therefore Andie = fun. Or perhaps I did already know my feelings for her. When a relationship goes wrong it is hard to admit that you ever did love that person. It would be easier for me to think that I did not have true feelings for Andie. What I will admit however, and what I have to say for the sake of the story, is that, at the time, I truly believed that I loved her.

She did not answer me, but when I left the next day, while I was on the train back, she text me 'I love you too'.

I had been given a reason to live. This one thing had saved me by having this person to love, by being loved in return. However, I couldn't relax and I couldn't believe that anything was better. It was just too surreal. I went to work but shirked my duties in favour of e-mailing or texting Andie. I thought about her all the time. I really believed that we were in a relationship and so I made a date to see her again.

Work had started a shift pattern that enabled us to get more orders out per day. The late shift was one o'clock in the afternoon until midnight. It was strange. I stayed in bed most of the morning and then I would cycle to the shop to get a bottle of cider to put in the fridge awaiting my return from work, as the shop wouldn't be open by the time I finished. Sometimes I would buy cans of beer and I took them to work with me. Michael and I would sit outside having a break and we would drink them chatting about music or our love lives. The warmth of summer air made working late seem almost exotic. I quite liked doing that shift. We brought CDs in and listened to them all night singing along as we did the menial task of scanning out clothing and putting it in boxes. It was so easy it hardly felt like work and having Michael there always helped. We always managed to talk to each other and have a laugh or seriously talk about our feelings; there was no macho front between us two.

I remember a text message I got from Andie while working late one night. It said 'I can't wait to see you again - I love you so much!' There were no obvious danger signs so I just kept going on the same road. I was heading down the road at great speed by now, not looking behind me. How was I to know the twists and turns that were ahead?

I guess the first sign came when she changed her mind about coming to my house. We had e-mailed and set up the visit for Saturday but on Saturday morning I got a strange e-mail from her saying she didn't think it was a good idea after all. I had allowances for her, knowing that she was like me and didn't find it easy to be sociable but I really wanted to see her - I guess I just needed some reassurance that this was a real relationship. I sent her a message straight back saying that I really wanted her to come, I had bought her a bottle of gin and we could just listen to music and get drunk; 'slagging' off the world. It took a further two e-mails to persuade her.

She came to Letchworth and I met her at the station. She seemed fine. She was smiling and gave me a hug and then we got a taxi to my house. It felt strange having her there; I guess she felt strange to be there too. She had brought some CDs with her and she had a good look through my collection and put some on. It should have been fine. We were drinking and chatting quite easily but I realised something; I realised that I never felt comfortable around Andie. I felt that I had to be a better Steve than I really was, that I had to put on a face. I wondered if it was just me, if I would feel that way about everyone, but then I thought I knew why I felt that way about Andie. I had put her on a pedestal and she was sitting so high on it that I was always looking up. I would never be able to reach her now and I didn't reach her all night.

We got drunk and went upstairs and put more music on. I felt very nervous, worried that she might expect sex, but really I think that it was I that was expecting it. This was my girlfriend after all, wasn't it? It didn't seem like she was mine, it seemed like I was borrowing her. She lay back on the bed and before I had a chance to notice she was asleep. Something was wrong here. I was in bed with a girl but this was definitely not my girlfriend.

The next morning Andie was very withdrawn and didn't seem to want to stay. I asked her to stay just a little while but she was determined to go home. What had I done or said to make her reject me like this? How could she say she loved me and then not want to spend time with me? I guessed she was just feeling depressed and so I had to be understanding, I took her back to the station and said my good byes. I was left feeling very confused and as I walked back home, I sank further and further back into my depression with every step I took. I began to remember the despair that only she was keeping away. Without her I would be more alone than I was before I met her. Now I had met her I couldn't bear to not know her.

I got home and I went back to bed, listening to a Morrissey CD my mind going crazy with maybes. I wondered if she had just realised that I was ugly. I wondered if she had just changed her mind and she didn't love me after all. Perhaps she had realised that I was too boring for her...Perhaps, perhaps, perhaps. I couldn't stop going over it all in my mind and I started to wonder why I bothered with girls. Girls always equalled pain to me yet I was so lonely and miserable, that it seemed a girlfriend would have to be the thing to save me. Kill or cure. With me that phrase is meant literally.

There was an e-mail waiting for me when I got to work on Monday morning.

'Steve, I don't think it's a good idea for us to be together. I can't do it. We are too much alike. Two depressed people together are not healthy. I'm sorry. Please be my friend. Andie.'

I felt like I had been punched in the stomach. What could I do to make this different? Couldn't I somehow go back in time, replay Saturday and convince her to love me? For she had said it hadn't she? She had said that she loved me and now this. Well it seemed that she had made her

162

mind up before Saturday hadn't she? She never wanted to come in the first place. I felt so gutted, so desperate because I had nothing now, no hope for the future, no will to live. Just as Carey had once saved me, Andie was to be her replacement, but now she was saying that she didn't want the job. There was no one and nothing else.

I went on with my work but my head wasn't with it, my brain was working overtime trying to compile a message to Andie that would change her mind. I hid away from any jobs, losing myself in the corners of the warehouse where no one was working, or spending hours in the toilets where I cut my arm up with a blade that I kept for that very reason. Michael noticed my mood and asked if I was all right, I was obviously acting as broken as I felt inside. I hadn't spoken a word to anyone and merely grunted at anyone that said hello or good morning. It wasn't a good morning it was a fucking terrible morning. Did these people not have bad things happen to them? Why were they always so fucking happy? At least Michael understood, he at least, had feelings. I told him and he seemed really sorry. He had seen how happy Andie had made me and now he could see how totally devastated I was.

I was scribbling on a bit of paper I carried around with me all day, writing declarations of love and arguments as to why two depressed people were perfect for each other. I would never mention the suicide pact, the twisted idea I had that I wanted someone to be miserable with. I realised there was one major difference between Andie and me and that was what kept us apart. Andie wanted to get better. I just wanted to die.

I sat at my desk in my lunch break and typed up the scribbled note into something that resembled sense. I read it back to myself. God I sounded desperate, but that was exactly what I was. I couldn't cope with this knock back, after hardly any time the thing I wanted was being taken away. I think I made up my mind then. I would try to get

163

Andie back but if I couldn't I would make a new date for my suicide and I would just get on and do it. I'd had enough of waiting around, waiting for a sign that reads 'do it now'. There is never going to be a good time to do it. It doesn't matter whether you have had a long drawn out depression or just a little set back; suicide is final and is a rejection of the world no matter when you do it. I had been putting it off in case something good happened, and now it had and it was over and I would wait no more.

Before I went home that night Andie had sent me another e-mail. I hardly dared to read it and clenched my teeth, breathing deeply through my nose. I opened it. I read it quickly, and then again slowly. There was no change. She was sticking by everything she had said and she was really sorry for hurting me but that was it, and she really wants me as a friend. I wanted to cry, but I waited until I got home. I went to the shop first of course, getting some cider to see me through the evening. What was I waiting for now? Should this not be the sign that I should kill myself? I sat and wrote in my diary that I would do it on October 1st that I would take an overdose of my antidepressants. I was set on it. Then I went upstairs and spent two hours rolling on my bed sobbing, punching the wall to take out my anguish and to hurt myself. Sobbing and saying "Why? Why can't I get what I want just once?" My life was a fucking Smiths record.

Despite my pain I somehow lived to see another day. I didn't go to work because I couldn't bear trying to act normal when inside I was a wreck. I stayed at home drinking and I cut up my arms. This had hit me and hit me hard. I had let down my defences and let someone in and this is what I got. I had lost all faith in life.

Time might be the great healer but it left you with scars. A month went by, weeks went on and Andie was still in contact over text messages, each one a kick in the teeth. I didn't give up though. Andie wanted me as a friend so I would be her friend and then, in time, perhaps we would get back together. …But there is nothing quite as hopeless as hope. I guess it kept me alive. The unfounded hope and wish to get back with Andie was a reason to keep putting off my death. The scheduled date of my death came and went without event. I wrote in my diary again and made a new date. I just wanted to give it a bit longer to see if Andie would come round although I didn't even know if that would stop me, but I knew from experience that things could get better. Things could change from one day to the next. I had survived suicide attempts already and if I had died I would never have seen the Cure, I would never have even met Andie. Perhaps that wouldn't have been such a bad thing. To love and to have lost is a damn sight worse than never to have loved at all. Whoever made up that original phrase is obviously happily married to his child hood sweetheart.

It was around this time that I saw something on the news about Seroxat. It was reporting on the fact that a high number of people experienced increased urges to self-harm while on the drug. I was cutting myself a lot and I was thinking about suicide, my diary was full of plans to end my existence. It was enough to scare me and some of the side effects were distressing me too. I got it into my head that I wanted to be taken off the meds and given something else. It certainly wasn't working and now I felt that it was probably making me worse. During the next appointment I had with the psychiatrist I told him what I wanted and he agreed to take me off the drug, which I would have to do gradually, and he prescribed me a new medication. I was given Mirtazapine, Zispin, which he said would also help the anxiety I had about leaving the house. I had told him of my anguish getting away from the mirror in the morning but I did not tell him much about my face problem. I never told anyone about that, it was too embarrassing and, I thought, had little to do with my mental state.

I went on the internet to look up this new medication but it was all in jargon that I could not understand. It is a tetracyclic piperazino-azepine that enhances central noradrenergic and serotonergic activity by blocking alpha-receptors in the brain. What I did find out was that it was of a different group to Seroxat and was often given as a second or third line antidepressant. They had tried me on the Seroxat and this was their next choice. I had moved a little further up the ladder of insanity.

I was to take 15mg a day for a week and then increase it to 30mg once I had stopped the Seroxat. There were no noticeable side effects from the new pills and the sexual side effects I had experienced with Seroxat had gone away. I felt I had done the right thing getting off that drug, but my thoughts of suicide did not go away. What had I actually got to live for? I was still in contact with Andie but even if she wanted to be with me I was too much of a head case to go on with it. Suicide, planned and written in my diary, was becoming a fore gone conclusion.

Andie asked me to go to see a band with her in London and so I went. It wasn't a good idea yet I was clinging to the hope that she had changed her mind about me. We went to the venue and it was awkward at first, I did not know how to go on with this night, but we went to stand upstairs where we could get a good view and I tried putting my arm around her. She let me do it.

"Do you mind me putting my arm around you?"

"No of course not," she said smiling back at me. I wondered what was going on here. I didn't feel at all comfortable but I kept my arm where it was. Perhaps I should be making a move. Perhaps she had changed her mind.

"Can I kiss you?"

"Steve, we're just friends remember."

I took my arm away and I sank into myself, shrivelling away, feeling completely trapped in my body. I wanted to die right then and there. I wanted to put an end to this alienation and the only reason I could think of for this continued rejection was that Andie did not find me attractive. I could hardly blame her. Perhaps she didn't like men that wore make up. Perhaps she found my innocence a turn off. Perhaps all those things had put Carey off me too. Perhaps I was completely wrong for Andie but how could it be that I was wrong for her and she was right for me? I didn't think it was supposed to work like that. That's what I couldn't work out.

We went our separate ways in the tube tunnels, I hugged her good bye, and I knew then that I would never see her again. I knew that I had a date with suicide.

You can't blame Andie. You shouldn't give her the credit for something that had been brewing up for months before hand. Blaming Andie is like blaming the shop that sells the paracetomol that some messed up kid takes all at once. Blaming Andie is like blaming Marilyn Manson for the fact that two of his fans went on a rampage through their school in Columbine. Blaming Andie would only be sensible if everything else was right with my life, but nothing was right in my life because I was depressed. …And I was depressed with being so miserable. I was drinking heavily, I was hiding from the world, the only world I had any part of was work and that was not through choice. More and more I would take days off so that I didn't have to put the make up on or because I had put the make up on and I still looked terrible. All too often going in to work was a trauma I just couldn't bear. I had a hang up about sex, a hang up about my own lack of intelligence. I had got nowhere with my writing and didn't know why I bothered anymore. I didn't know why I bothered with anything in my life. I didn't enjoy half the things I used to hold dear. Even music seemed futile to me. So blaming Andie is not going to give you an answer as to

167

why I felt suicidal. If it weren't her that triggered me it would only have been something or someone else.

I got home from work on Monday night and lay on my bed writing my next diary entry on a page of lined paper.

'Dear diary,

I am in love with misery, constantly embracing death, yet as with any love it bears such a resemblance to hate. ...But happiness is an alien thing to me and after years of seeking it, its poison now runs through my veins and threatens to kill me. All those years waiting for pleasure's taste only to find it bitter. It was not worth waiting for.

...And so I will not wait much longer. I lay here allowing misery to fill my room, resigning myself to this life. I am ill, I know, but there is no cure. I can only get better by allowing myself that which I have put off for so many years, and I may never know that it has worked.

I lay here knowing that I have only days left; yet I have no urgency to move. There is nothing I need to do before I go, only Tuesday, yet Wednesday's task is as sure as it has ever been. I have, at last, set myself a fixed date to descend into the darkness that has always been trying to suck me in. I have nothing left to fight with and I am tired of the struggle. Why struggle anyway? Why hope when all hope is lost? Why stay when I find no pleasure in any of it? It is as much as I can do to put it off these last few days- so set am I.

Yet I fear one thing - I fear failure because failure has lasted so long. I want to go this time, I have no hope left.'

168

I don't remember why I picked that Wednesday. Perhaps I had a few things to put into place first. Perhaps I just wanted a few clear days to get my head around it, to experience the pleasure of knowing that I didn't have to put up with life much longer. ...But the date was set for Wednesday and Wednesday soon came.

I acted perfectly normal. I went to work and did my job. Everyone was used to me being withdrawn; they wouldn't have noticed any change. They may have noticed, however, by my choice of CD, that this was one of my bad days.

"This is depressing music." You don't say... Then maybe I'm depressed; did you ever think of that one? I had made myself two complete tapes of dark, beautiful songs that I could play on my last night. Suicide tape one and suicide tape two.

My depression had gone back to the way it was before and had gone way past being anything to do with Andie. Yes it still hurt that she had rejected me, yes it stung every time she text messaged me or sent me an e-mail, but I had resigned myself to the fact that she didn't want me. Weeks went by and I accepted it more and more, yet she was still in my life sending messages to refuel any feelings I had for her and to mess me up again.

'My heart ignores the danger signs. I go out of my way for this pain. I chase it, call it, text it, and then it is mine...but only for a moment. Yet I never forget a moment.'

I thought that I was Pip from Great Expectations, doomed to love this girl for no real reason yet it would destroy my whole life, all the time waiting for her to choose to be with me. That seemed like the most romantic way to look at it. It would have been closer to the truth that she was a witch come to mess me up. Well I wasn't going to let her spoil my death.

Wednesday was a day of dark twisted thoughts and of hiding from sight. I went to the toilet a lot just to stand and stare at my reflection, looking to see if you could actually see the darkness that surrounded me. Then, the evening came and I went to Sainsbury's and did some shopping, mainly because I needed alcohol, walking around the shop as though I were in a bubble, trapped in there with my thoughts and the little black cloud that always hovered above my head. Today was the day; remember? Why was I bothering to buy food? ...But there I was walking around with a basket, heavy with cider, thinking about what I might like to eat that week.

...And then I went to pay for it and I looked at everyone there, people living their lives, not for a second thinking about killing themselves or looking at me and seeing death behind my eyes. No one would guess that this was my last night on Earth; no one would really care. All those people that had decided to shop at the same time as me; all those people that had nothing else in common with me than the day and time they were doing their shopping. All those people, the last people to see me alive. It felt unreal. I imagined a bomb dropping on the shop and wiping them all out and me with them.

Then, I rode home, tasting the twilight air, making my last ever journey. I put my bike in the garden, I couldn't be bothered to open the garage, and I checked on my rabbit. She seemed fine, she had no idea what I was doing and so long as she had food and water she wouldn't care. I filled her bowl with food and stroked her a little.

170

"Good-bye bunny," I whispered.

When I got in I put the shopping away as I would always do and put the cider in the fridge, then I went online. No important e-mails, nothing that was going to stop me going through with my plan. No declarations of love, but would that even have saved me at this point? I don't know. Perhaps I just had enough reasons to do it now. Perhaps I was only waiting until I had a full list of reasons. Perhaps nothing would have stopped me. I wasn't thinking about anyone, I was thinking about myself and the life I had to endure everyday. I was thinking about my desire to just not be here. I was thinking about the fact that nothing good ever lasts and is never that great anyway. The fact that I worked in a dull warehouse all day with people that only pretended to be my friends, having to see them no matter how I felt inside. ...And then there was my skin, the awful suffocating phobia I had about people seeing what I really looked like.

I thought about the sky, about tigers, about swimming in the sea and about everything this world has to offer and I just thought... "It's just not enough. None of it is enough to keep me here". ...And I thought about my music and my writing and I just thought, "Well if I'm dead then none of that will matter anyway. So what have I got to lose?" I thought that perhaps when I died my book would get published and maybe, just maybe, from what ever after life I have I might see it. Famous when you're dead. I could be a cult.

I went on to the forums that I sometimes used. There was the Tori Amos forum but that also linked to forums about other things. I went on to the one about depression and suicidal thoughts. I wanted to spill my guts, tell everyone what I was doing and how I was feeling. ...Why did I want to do that? I just didn't want to be alone with this, and I felt more alone than I had ever felt in my life. There was nothing and no one to stop me this time. I didn't want the users of the forum to read my message and start

171

telling me how I had everything to live for. What did they know anyway? They didn't know me and that's what was good about writing on there, it was completely anonymous.

'I've decided to do it tonight. I can't put it off any longer and why should I wait just because I had set a date? What is to stop me doing it right now? There is nothing in my life to live for because none of it matters. It's not easy to explain what's wrong with me. If you just look at the sum of the parts, it doesn't add up to much. Yet I feel pretty desperate and at the same time, quite numb. It's like I am not really living. I never have been. It's like I'm constantly waiting for something to happen, something to kick-start my existence. I want something to live for, but instead I just find more reasons why it is pointless. I am fed up with waiting. I actually feel like I'm going to be too old soon to start living.

There's a girl that I wanted to be with and she doesn't want to be with me... fair enough, it sucks but I could get over it - except that my whole life is like that. Every time I think it's going to happen for me it gets thrown back in my face as if it was all a sick joke. The things I want are a million miles away and the things I don't want are here on a plate. I am constantly having it proven to me that life and hope is futile.

On top of that, everyday I see or hear something that makes me despair at the world. I see how people act and they make me sick. Like the guys at work all making sexual jokes and never thinking any deeper than football. I feel too fragile to be on this planet - too emotional, too weak, too fucked up, too ugly, too socially inept. I try to think of positive things but the negatives just stamp them into the ground.

I should probably just get on with life but how can I when I don't have the coping mechanisms that other people have. All I do with my life is drink and imagine myself sitting on the train tracks. I don't want to live in my fantasy world any more; I want to live the dream. That means I have to die.'

I posted the message and then I e-mailed Carey and told her that she would not be hearing from me again as I was going to kill myself. I guess I thought I owed her that much.

Then I turned off the computer. It felt good to get it out there, to put my feelings into words, but I wasn't interested in reading any replies. I was sure that I was going to do it; I was going to take an overdose. My chest was tight and I breathed deeply through my open mouth. Think, what do I need to do before I go? I was thinking perfectly rationally, except that I was thinking myself into an early grave. I knew that I had to tell someone what I had done so that they could find my body before it starts to rot. It was a gross thought but it made sense. I couldn't let my mother find me after I had been dead for days.

My social worker was due to come the next day so I wrote a note to him.

'I have taken an overdose please get help.'

...But it wasn't help I wanted; it was an end to my perpetual pain, to the enduring hopelessness, and to the incessant death wish. I just wanted to go.

I taped the note to the front door and stood looking at it for a moment watching it flap in the wind. Then I went

173

back inside, got the cider from the fridge, took a glass and went upstairs.

I put in suicide tape one and the gentle music started. This was my last night on Earth so was I thinking about whether there was anything I wanted to do before I died? Was I thinking about whether I had any regrets about my life? No. I didn't even think like that. I didn't care that I was soon going to be dead. I didn't care that I hadn't seen America. I didn't care that I would never see my family again. I didn't care what people would think of me. My rational thoughts had left me and left me with one aim - to commit suicide. It wasn't romantic or even particularly cathartic; it was just something that I was going to do. This was the end of my life and that was the best thing that could happen all round. My family would be upset but they would get over it - it was only me remember. I was always the black sheep in the family, the miserable one that had tried to kill himself. Well now I was going to put an end to all that.

I was scared though. I thought that I had enough pills to kill myself with but I didn't know how my body would react and how exactly they would kill me. I didn't know if there would be any pain. I just wanted to sleep and not wake up. I wrote in the note pad by the bed, putting down the time and my thoughts. I hoped that my mother and other members of my family would read my last words and perhaps understand it better. I knew it would be hard for them but if they could just get into my mind a little they might realise that I had no choice.

'7.30.

Tonight is the night that I end it all. I am sorry, but I cannot go on. I cannot live with this depression any longer. My mind has always incarcerated my happiness in a cage it

174

could never escape from and now I finally get my peace. I am so sorry, I love you all.'

    I started drinking from the glass, listening to the music and sitting upright on my bed. So this is where it would end. These are the last songs I would hear. It was just as I wanted it to be.

    I opened the drawer in the bedside cabinet and took out all the blister packs of tablets I had in there. I had only recently picked up the prescription and so I had just under a month's supply. I put them all on the bed and sat there looking at them. I forgot how difficult it was to pluck up the courage to take them, and I guessed that I would have to get drunk first. I had a mirror in the cabinet and I took that out and looked at myself. That was enough to make me feel like dying. I still had the days make up on and during the course of all those hours it had begun to dry and look more obvious. I decided not to wash it off in case I ended up in hospital. That was what was different about taking an overdose compared with other ways to kill yourself: With an overdose there is always the chance that you might survive. It was in the hands of the Gods. It was either my destiny to die or my destiny to fail and to be treated in hospital. ...But I had made provisions for either situation and I welcomed both. So I turned over the tape and I drank some more.

'8.45.

    The drink is working its magic and I am getting quite drunk. What I am going to do seems so easy yet I still fear it. I am set in my mind though; this is the end of my life.'

175

...And then I drank some more and I popped all the pills out onto the bed. I remembered the last overdose I had taken and I remembered doing this then. So this is how it's done. This is how you go about ending your life. Some people had never experienced such things. To some people this would not even cross their minds, yet it crossed mine every day. Now, at last, I was doing something about it. Now that I had no hope that I would ever be happy I was ready to accept my fate.

'9.30.

I have taken the pills. I am terrified of what might happen to me but I plucked up the courage and I took them. Now I must wait and sleep and hope to never wake. Please don't feel bad for me. This is what I wanted. I'm sorry.'

...And the last thing I remember was laying down on my bed holding the mirror at arms length from my face, what I thought would be the last time I would ever look at myself, and I dropped the mirror on the bed beside me and shut my eyes.

I heard a knocking at the door but all I could see was darkness and felt something soft against my face. I tried to move but my whole body seemed paralysed. I tried to move my legs and they were heavy but moved a little in one sudden jolt. I couldn't remember anything that explained this paralysis; I didn't think about what I had done;

I didn't really think at all. I just tried to move. There was a voice but I couldn't place it, I couldn't think who it was or why it was or from where it was coming from. I lifted my head and it rolled back on my neck and then dropped back down into the softness that was a pillow. Somehow I managed to roll onto my back and my open eyes swam a blurred view of the ceiling. I sat up straight and the room revolved around me, the bed like a magic carpet flying over some strange land. I clung on to the bed lest I fall.

The bed was covered in tablet packaging and there was the mirror I always kept close by. I picked it up and tried to look at myself but I couldn't keep my hands steady and my reflection was fuzzy and kept moving. I dropped it back down. I remembered what I had done now. I remembered that I was supposed to be dead and I knew that I had failed and that I somehow had to live through this and get some help. The knocking at the door must have been my social worker. This was the day after the night before, the day that wasn't supposed to come.

I put my feet on the floor and stood up. I fell forwards and put my hands out to grab something, clutching hold of the open door and trying to make my feet follow. Somehow I stayed upright; somehow I was at the top of the stairs.

The voice came again.

"Stephen can you hear me?"

It was a man's voice, it didn't take long to place it, it was Owen, my social worker.

I was at the top of the stairs and I knew I had to try and get down them, but it felt like all my bones had turned to jelly. I had no strength in my legs and I could only stay upright by leaning against the painted wall. I slid down and sat on the first step and began to slide slowly down. I could see my front door and could see a figure behind the glass. Then, as I got further down, the letterbox opened and my name was called through it.

"Stephen can you here me?" It was a different voice.

When I got to the bottom step I put my hand on the banister and tried to stand. My whole body was tingling as if it were being gently electrocuted. Pins came into my hand as I tightened my grip on the wooden banister and used what little strength I had to pull myself up.

I could see more figures behind the door now and blue flashing lights that must have been an ambulance. I often wonder how long it would have taken them to break the door down, but there I was, tuning the key in the lock.

I fell back against the wall just as I caught sight of the ambulance staff and Owen all moving towards me. They put out there hands and they grabbed me gently about the waist leading me out the door. They were speaking they were asking me things but I couldn't focus.

"What did you take Stephen?"

"My antidepressants." I slurred, my voice coming out in waves, my mouth dry and uncoordinated.

"Is that the Mirtazapine?"

"Yes." It was too difficult to concentrate on talking; I only hoped they wouldn't ask me anything else.

I was still fully dressed; I was even wearing a pair of sneakers. Just as well because I didn't have the energy or the sense to get myself ready. I worried about locking my

178

house but Owen was taking care of that. I think he said something about my mum but she wasn't there. This was still my little secret, yet I couldn't bear to keep this to myself, it was too much of a burden. I wanted everyone to know and I wanted to be looked after. ...And that was what was happening. I was being taken into the ambulance and I was lying on the stretcher. It felt so good to be lying down again. The toil of getting out of bed and down those stairs had really taken it out of me. Lying down my mind relaxed and my eyesight steadied. I could see the people that were there to help me and there they were, helping me, taking my blood pressure, talking to each other about me.

At the hospital I did not have my stomach pumped and I was not sick. I think I had slept through that stage and now it was too late. I didn't know if I had done myself any major damage. They did their tests, took my blood and I was laying there waiting for the ill affects to die off, waiting for them to give me the all clear, waiting to speak to a psychologist or a psychiatrist no doubt. The nurses hadn't asked why I did it but I guess they could see from my notes that I had a history. I did it because I was depressed. I did it because life sucks and offers no hope for betterment. I did it because I could.

I was in the hospital all alone for hours. I kept checking my watch and thinking how work must be wondering where I was, but I had no way of contacting them. I wondered if Owen would tell my mother. I wondered if that's what I heard him say. Perhaps he had asked me if he should. Perhaps I had said no and that's why I was here, abandoned, and left in a cubicle with nothing but my own thoughts. I wished that it had worked. I wished that I didn't have to be there facing this day. Then I saw the face of my mother and my sister, those weary expressions of pain and puzzlement.

"Steve," my mother said as she made her way to my bedside. She looked as if she was going to cry. "What are

179

you doing back here again; I thought you weren't going to do this anymore." She came close and held my tingling hand. My sister came to the other side of me and just gave me a loving smile. How could I explain to my family why I had done it again? How could I tell them that their love is just not enough to keep me here? My family life was just not a big enough slice to make it all better. There was my love life, my work life and my home life - that was how I spent most of my hours; hours, days and weeks in despair. If I had died then my family would no doubt get over it, move on, and Andie, Carey, Michael and perhaps even Rick and Dave would be dressed in black and singing my praises.

We were all waiting now, my family around me trying to make me feel better, trying to act calm even after what I had done. My mother told me that Owen had left an urgent message on her phone asking her to call him back, but she hadn't got the message until she got back home from work. By then it was too late and Owen and the other mental health workers had all gone home. She had to ring the hospital in fear that I was there and they had told her I was and that I was going to be ok. Then my father and his wife appeared and they greeted me with a smile, smiling only for my sake, and I recoiled on my bed, wanting them there, but not wanting to ever know what I had done to them.

I went to the toilet, managing to walk although I dragged my feet. I urinated, the very act of it seeming miraculous and making me feel that some of the poison that was in my body had been drained. Then I got to the mirror and stared at my face. It looked bright red, and it felt like it was burning. Most if not my entire make up, had rubbed off and I had some new beard growth on my chin. Here I was, looking my worst and all of my family was out there, all of them looking at me. I worried that they might be thinking how ugly I was. I wondered if I was a disappointment to my mother and father because, although I was fairly good looking my skin was spoilt.

180

I did something then that I never dared to do when I had no make up close at hand. I ran my hands under the cold tap, cupped them to catch the water and threw the water against my face, cooling my burning cheeks. I figured I looked awful anyway so a bit of water wasn't going to hurt. I tried to wet my hair down a little too, trying to make the most of a spoilt canvas and at that point my dad came in.

"Handsome devil aren't you boy?" He said.

It wasn't his fault. He had no idea that I wanted to curl up in a ball and hide just so that no one could see this 'handsome' face. He had no idea that being so unhandsome was one of the core reasons I had done this in the first place. We went back to the cubicle together and I got back on the bed feeling worse now that I had seen myself and wishing that I would have some freak reaction to the overdose that suddenly stopped my heart. I wondered if I looked as bad to them as I did to myself.

Eventually, the psychiatrist and someone else that introduced himself as a psychologist saw me. They asked if I wanted anyone with me and I said that I wanted to see them alone. I could tell them the truth but I wasn't going to tell my family the ins and outs of my brain. Only I knew my real reasons and they didn't even make sense to me. Perhaps they would make sense to a professional.

I told them how I had wanted to die since I was a child and that I just didn't want this so called 'gift'. I told them that every time I think that something is going right for me it gets thrown back in my face. I told them that my nose was red and my skin was thin and disgusting and I couldn't live looking like this. I told them that my life was not worth living and that I was disappointed to not be dead. I basically told him every reason I had ever had and every one of those reasons was the reason that I did it. The doctor asked me some more straightforward questions, the old spiel that I would soon get very used to. Then he asked me something that really knocked some sense into me.

"Do you think it would help you to spend some time with us, in the ward?"

They wanted to put me away! This was serious. They wanted to know if I thought I was crazy enough to be in the mental health ward. I thought about it briefly, wondering whether it would be worth it for the experience, wondering if a rest from life would improve things for me. I wondered if perhaps this was how my life was supposed to turn out. ...But to be put on the ward with more depressed people, with people who really were insane; I couldn't see how that would benefit me.

"No, I just want to go home."

"Well how likely do you feel it is that you might do something like this again?"

It was very likely. Not in the near future as I felt too ill and as always the idea of doing anything more to my body frightened me, but it was very likely that I would kill myself one day because that was how I was destined to die. I would try it again and next time I would do it right.

"I don't want to do it again."

"Ok then. If we can trust you then I think we can let you go, but have you got someone you can stay with for a while?"

"I can probably stay with my mum."

"Ok, then do that. Ok take care of yourself Stephen."

And that was it - I had passed the sanity exam despite the fifty odd pills I had taken last night. I was a free man - just.

My mother said that I should come to hers before I even mentioned it and my dad said I could stay with him if I would rather, but for some reason I chose my mother's. I guess I just knew that she would leave me alone a little more than my father would have done. They wouldn't leave me alone long enough to try something again though, that was for sure. I had become high risk as well as high maintenance.

Dark Little Secrets

I got some things from my house, including my make up, and I went with my mother to her house. I stayed there for one night and spent the whole time wishing I were alone. She was frightened when she came back to my house, frightened to leave me, frightened because I had now tried to kill myself three times. I think I really frightened my family with this latest attempt; I think it helped them see the seriousness of my condition and helped them see my mortality. I was severely depressed and it could possibly be terminal.

I remember my mother wanted to stay for a while before she felt good enough to leave me on my own. We decided to watch a movie together first.

I went upstairs where I kept my videos and DVDs and I went into the bedroom. It was just as I had left it with the rubbish from the pills all over the bed and the mirror there that I always kept in the bedside cabinet. I wished that I could have a normal depression rather than the one I had. I wished that I didn't put so much emphasis on what I looked like and I wished that I could look in the mirror without going into a state of panic. I picked up the mirror and held it up to myself in the semi dark room. I looked as I always looked. I threw the mirror down onto the cabinet and it cracked in half.

"Shit." I said under my breath. Seven more years bad luck then, as if I would notice the difference. I also realised that I hadn't got any of my medication left so I would have to go to the doctors tomorrow. Everything was too much trouble and I didn't want any of it. My mother's presence was irritating me as well. I wanted to be alone and get on the internet and speak to people on the forum. I wondered if anyone had answered my last post. I would have to tell them I was ok, that I was still alive, and they would all think that was such a good thing. My virtual world seemed more important or perhaps just easier to deal with.

Eventually my mother went and I was alone. It felt strange and it didn't feel safe. I could do something to myself; I knew it. I knew I wasn't far from that peak despite having carried it out days ago. The only thing that would stop me thinking of death was to be dead and I wished that my overdose had worked.

It was quite late but I had every intention of drinking what was left of the cider and checking things online.

I had an e-mail from Carey, a condemning message that went along the lines of 'I don't believe you are ever going to kill yourself, stop attention seeking and just get on with your life. You are a young, nice and good looking guy, you'll find someone one day.' I took offence at the fact that she hadn't taken me seriously. I was annoyed that she thought the only reason I did it was loneliness and rejection. There was much more involved than that, but how could I expect her to understand? She had never been interested enough to work me out. I sent her a reply telling her that I did in fact do what I had threatened to do, but that I was alive and well and putting my life back together thank you very much. As I wrote it I realised that I didn't believe a word of it. My life was in pieces and they didn't even fit together anymore. I had survived another attempt at my life but I knew it wouldn't be the last. It just wasn't as cathartic as I thought it would be.

I had replies to my forum post. They were quite sincere and caring despite the fact that those people didn't really know me. ...But they had read my post and they had bothered to reply, trying to talk me out of it when all the time they had no chance because I had just turned off the computer. I read them all and then replied.

'Thank you for your concern. I did take an overdose but I am still alive and kicking and trying to live my life again in the aftermath. It's never easy to pick yourself up, going back to the same old life that you tried to escape from, but I will certainly try. Thanks again.'

The next day I went to the doctor's. I had no intention of going to work and why should I? I was ill. You might not be able to see depression but that doesn't make it any less real. If I had a broken leg, I wouldn't be expected to work yet I am supposed to just pick myself up after nearly dying a few days ago. I didn't care what my boss thought about it, but I figured that I owed him the truth. Perhaps if work knew why I had so much time off, they might be sympathetic. I knew that I was skating on thin ice and could be in danger of getting sacked, but if they knew I was ill perhaps I could get away with it. The world and its ideas were supposed to be advanced and modern weren't they? Depression never used to be understood but now it was quite common. I didn't like to think of that, to know it was nothing special. I wanted to be special. No one could have ever been through what I had been through. No one felt like I felt. My depression was serious. If it were the sixties, I would probably have been put away for my suicide attempts. I would probably be given electric shock treatment. Perhaps that's what I needed to get death out of my mind.

I didn't see my own doctor, I saw a lady instead. The doctor made me out a prescription for my meds and she asked me how I was. I told the truth, that I still felt shell shocked and dreaded having to go to work and try to act normal.

"We wouldn't expect you to go straight back to work after this. You haven't even had chance to come to terms with what you did. I will sign you off for a month and then you can try to get back to normality. Ok?"

Yes, that's what I needed. I needed a break. Perhaps needing a break was the only reason I had tried to kill myself in the first place. I would have to tell work though. I would tell my boss the truth and hope that he keeps it from everyone else. I didn't want the guys I worked with to treat me differently or talk about me behind my back. I wondered if they had sort of guessed anyway. Perhaps my insanity was glaringly obvious.

I rode back up the road towards my house and called in at work.

"Hello stranger." I was greeted with puzzled expressions.

I was shaking at the thought of having to tell my dark secrets to someone that I had to see each day and I had no idea what his reaction would be. Perhaps he would want to sack me for having all this time off. Perhaps it was not their policy to allow a member of staff to have a whole month off. A month did, in fact, sound like a long time.

"Keith, I need to talk to you."

"Ok, take a seat."

I shut the office door and sat in front of my boss. I hated looking at him because his skin was always pale and blemish free. I worked quite closely with him and had to look at his face all the time. I knew that he didn't wear make up, you could tell, you could see each pore. I wondered how obvious my make up was. I looked at everyone's skin, comparing it to mine and wishing it were. I wondered if people looked as closely at me.

"I've been to the doctor's this morning and I've been signed off for a month."

"Ok," he wanted me to go on.

"The truth is that I suffer with depression. I took an overdose."

"Oh." He tried not to look surprised. "Are you ok?"

"A little shell shocked, hence the time away. I find it hard being with people."

"Yes of course. Is this anything to do with the other times you have been away or been late?"

"Yes, most of it has been mental. I find it hard to leave the house some mornings; I get panicky."

"Well I have noticed that sometimes, when you come in late you are a little bit 'rabbit in the head lights' for the first hour or so."

"I am taking medication but it doesn't seem to work."

"Are you seeing a psychologist or anything?"

"I'm supposed to be. I haven't started yet."

"Ok, well thank you for confiding in me, I will obviously keep this discreet but I may have to tell someone upstairs to keep them off your back."

The 'someone upstairs' meant the bosses above Keith. I realised there was no avoiding that, but I wondered how understanding they would be as they were obsessed with work and their careers and had no time for such things.

"Ok."

"Well take care of yourself, have a break and we will see you in a month ok?"

"Ok."

...And that was done with. I breathed the fresh air outside and for a moment felt very relieved and believed that I had my boss's support. Keeping down a job when you feel so utterly suicidal was not easy. So I wouldn't have to worry about that for four weeks, but what was I going to do with the time? I wondered if being alone for that long would actually help me. I wondered if I might be able to spend the entire month in bed letting my skin heal. Perhaps I would emerge completely cured. Or perhaps I would just get worse with all that time alone to think about things.

When I next saw my psychiatrist my mother insisted on coming with me. She wasn't happy at the way I was being treated; she thought that they were not doing enough to keep me safe. I kind of agreed with her, although I didn't know what else they could do. They had offered to have me in the ward and I had declined. I had said that I wanted to go it alone and that's exactly how it was.

My psychiatrist said that if I continued to overdose on a regular basis he would not be able to work with me anymore. I couldn't believe what he had said to me. He had said that if I become suicidal again and act on it he would no longer be my doctor. It sounded wrong. That couldn't have been what he meant, but he did. Perhaps it was just a scare tactic to make me tow the line. I don't know why he said it but neither my mother nor I thought it sounded very professional. If that were how he felt about it then I would get a second opinion. I asked to see a different doctor in future, would see the therapist as arranged, and would continue to see my social worker. My mother just wanted them to keep me from harm and I just wanted to die.

I had already started to write a skeleton plot for my next novel and had begun researching it. I had a book of mysterious creatures and I read some stories about fairies and became very interested in the old folk tales about them. It was good to read these old world myths, which painted a dark picture of these little creatures. They were evil, mischievous little things and I thought they deserved to have a novel written about them. This was the beginning of 'Dark Little Secrets', my second novel. This month off was a perfect time to write and to research it further. Writing was always a good way to occupy my mind when nothing else was going on but my inner misery. I went on the internet and searched for fairies, faeries, pixies and piskies and it all came clear through all this that Cornwall was their home. I would have to go to Cornwall and look for them.

I got quite excited at the thought of going to a strange place on my own and I hadn't had a holiday since my ill-fated wedding. It would be a perfect break from life, wandering around Cornwall, which I had heard was a beautiful place, and writing my novel. That's what a writer does, they research places by going there. I realised that I couldn't even start 'Dark Little Secrets' until I had been there. I wanted to go right then and there.

I am very proud of myself for what I did next. I surfed the internet for holidays to Cornwall and the name that kept coming up was Tintagel. There was a lot of mythology about the place, about King Arthur and piskies - the creatures that I had decided to write about. That was where I would have to go if I was going to be serious about this writing thing and I was serious. That's what I wanted most out of my fragile life. I wanted to be a writer and if my first novel hadn't made it then why not write another? …And if Tintagel was the place I had to go to research it, then that was where I would go.

I found hotels, bed and breakfast places and I found trains that went from London to Cornwall and I booked them all up for the following April. I wanted to go sooner but it was going to be an outside kind of holiday so I needed the better weather. I e-mailed the bed and breakfast place that I had booked with and asked if they knew any taxi numbers that could get me to them from the train station. There was no train directly to Tintagel. I was very proud of myself for doing all this and I was proud of myself for trying to live. Perhaps I would see how I got on with this novel and then make a decision about whether to live or not. This was another chance at happiness, something else to put my death off for. It was a good thing.

It was all booked up, the train, the taxi, the bed and breakfast, but now what? I was off work but once I had done all the research I could at home, I was left floundering. I had nothing to occupy myself with and spent days and days at home not seeing a soul. I didn't rest. I might lie on my bed for a while but then I would get up and go to the mirror. Or I would lie there holding up the shard of glass from my bedside mirror and search my face for blemishes. Seeing a little of it at a time was sometimes better, but before long I would be up and in the bathroom with my nose pressed up against the glass almost crying in despair. It was always on my mind and I lived in fear that I would need to go out or someone would knock on the door.

I stuck it for a week or so but I wasn't doing well. I was writing short prose occasionally but mostly I was just listening to music and feeling depressed. I couldn't see much point in my life. No one needed me. Although I was someone I was nobody's someone. There was no one in my life that would not be able to get over my death. Sure they would be upset for a little while but they would learn to live with it. No one's loss would be as great as mine. I had lost my will to live; I had lost it when I was a kid. I didn't know what was going to become of me in the long term. It wouldn't take much to tip me one way or the other and I was always teetering on the edge of forever. I guess I was hoping that my book would get published or someone would come and save me, but what I really needed was to not be ill any longer.

I asked my mother if I could live with her for a week. After the overdose I had wanted to be alone but now being alone was dangerous. I could see the danger signs; I knew them all too well now. I was writing things in my diary about wanting death, about what I wanted played at my funeral. I was looking up ways of committing suicide on the internet and there was a surprising amount of web sites telling you how to do it and what would happen if you did. It was quite sick really, and so was I.

My mother was scared because this request came out of the blue and was not in my nature, but I just knew that I shouldn't be left alone. I was in a dark place and couldn't really see the light. The only thing that kept me alive was thinking that perhaps I could wait until I had been to Cornwall. Maybe I could wait until I had written this novel and so she said that of course I could stay with her.

192

I was at my mum's and I was in a kind of daze the whole time. I couldn't really think or talk I just sat on a wooden stall at the back door watching the garden. I sat there for days watching the leaves change colour. ...But most of all I was watching a massive hornet fly around the bird box as if it wanted to get in it and make a nest. I made it a vendetta to kill the bloody thing. I was captain fucking Ahab sitting there, staking it out with a can of insecticide in my hand. That was all I cared about. I never really kill anything if I can help it yet I wanted to save my mother from having a whole nest of these giant wasps in her back garden. So I pursued this creature and as soon as I saw it I left my stall and went at it with the spray. It flew away and I watched it go up into the branches of the apple tree. So I went under the tree and looked up and there it was, on a branch, trying to wash the poison from its body. I would have felt sorry for it if I wasn't so set on its destruction. I sprayed it again.

This went on and on for a whole week. I sat there listening to the same CD that I had brought with me over and over and watching that damn hornet. Come the evening I shut the door and went inside. I would sit and watch the TV or a film on video and I sat on the sofa wishing that this wasn't my life, wishing that something would change.

Nothing really changed. Eventually I went back to work and no one asked where I had been. I guessed that they all knew or they didn't care, I didn't know what I would prefer. I was having a nightmare with my face all the time and I was feeling suicidal on a daily basis. I was seeing a psychologist in my lunch breaks and would spend over an hour talking about things with her and get back to work late. The boss knew where I was going and I promised to make up the time. I never did.

The therapist was a nice lady but she kept looking at me as if to say 'you really are in a mess aren't you?' I told her everything but none of it was anything I hadn't told

193

myself. I have always been introspective and just telling someone else about it wasn't going to make it go away. It was good to get it out there I suppose. I said that I thought, "Death would be easier", that "death is an easy option for me". I said, "The reasons for living are becoming clouded." I said, "I know I am going to kill myself." I didn't hold anything back and certainly didn't worry how this made the therapist feel. I told her how I felt like I was a nothing and only when I was part of a relationship did I feel I contributed something to life.

After a long session of talking about my problems in the past and my problems at the time, I left the therapist and went back to work. …But all that I had said and all that she had said, just stayed with me until the evening when I could get some cider drink the whole bottle and cut my arms with the broken mirror. That was my way of relieving my tension and the stress that dredging up all my problems had caused, but I guess it was a good idea for me to have a psychologist. When I felt particularly bad I could go there and tell her that I was having distressing thoughts. I couldn't tell anyone else that I was suicidal and I knew that I was thought of as a high risk of suicide. Strange that these people knew that about me, and my own family did not. I couldn't tell my mother or my father despite the fact that, since my last overdose, they phoned me every day to see how I was. I always just said that I was ok. I don't know if they believed me or not.

The psychologist started a therapy regime with me called 'cognitive therapy'. I was given work sheets to fill in and apparently this would help me turn negative thoughts 'I want to die' into positive ones 'I didn't mean it'. So I did it, I filled in the damn home work sheets. Situation, moods, automatic thoughts or images, evidence that supports the 'hot' thought, evidence that does not support the 'hot' thought, alternative balanced thoughts and mood rating at the end. It didn't help. How the hell could it help when I strongly believed that the main reason for my 'hot' thoughts was that I was right? I was ugly and I did want to die. I was depressed because the world was a crap place that held nothing for me but, pain, boredom and mediocrity. If I had been thinking this way ever since I was a child, how could filling in a few sheets change me? I was set like this for life and I wanted to end it. I was depressed, suffering anhedonia (apparently) and had a borderline personality disorder with features of chronic worries and depressive episodes. That's what the doctors wrote about me. It made me sound so important.

...But life goes on doesn't it? Unless you do something to stop it life just runs away with itself and before long you are thirty years old with a wife and two kids and a shitty job. I didn't want any of that, but I wanted something and so I lived.

Christmas came and I sat at my sister's house eating her food, drinking her beer and playing with the kids, but despair wasn't far from my mind. All of it just seemed so futile when you could just kill yourself. Everything in life is a waste of time because you are going to die one day, and if, like me, you were planning to go sooner rather than later, why bother doing anything? Christmas was always a let down. I maintain that I like Christmas, that it is the only good thing about winter and was, in fact, designed to make winter more bearable, but once it was over it left you with a hole. I told my sister that I was seeing Michael on New Year's night and I told Michael I was going to my sisters'. I locked the door, drew the curtains, lit candles and watched episodes of 'Buffy the vampire slayer' all alone, drinking myself into a numb apathy. I celebrated midnight with my rabbit and when the fireworks stopped I put her back in her hutch and went to bed.

April. This was the date of my holiday. I packed only a few changes of clothes, my writing pad, personal stereo and my toiletries. I packed my make up although I was kind of hoping not to use it. There wouldn't be anybody there that would ever see me again so what did it matter if they thought I had bad skin? Perhaps the sea air would help heal it? I packed it anyway.

I made the trip to London, and waited for my train that would take me to Bodmin. A tramp asked me for money and I took pity on him. I asked if he wanted the money for food and he said that he did so I said that I would not give him money, but that I would buy him a burger. He thanked me very much and staggered away to eat his Burger King in peace. I bought one for myself.

I enjoyed the train journey because it was the start of an adventure. I listened to my personal stereo, listening to my suicide tapes, and looked out of the window the whole time watching the city turn to countryside. It took hours to get there but I wasn't bored I was writing my novel in my head, thinking of the characters that would be my company during the trip. I was alone but it was my choice and I wouldn't have wanted anyone there with me. This wasn't so much a holiday as a voyage of self-discovery.

The taxi was waiting for me as soon as I arrived and another couple were sharing the ride with me. That meant that it would only cost me half as much. All was going according to plan. The rest of the journey went by jovially with the other couple chatting to the driver and with me silent in the back seat. I was itching to get there now and soon enough, after dropping off the couple at their hotel, I was driven a little further and arrived at my bed and breakfast by late afternoon.

I was greeted by the man that ran the place and went inside with him carrying my bag.

"So what brings you to Tintagel?" He asked me.

"I'm writing a novel," I said proudly, "I want to base it in Cornwall."

My room was small but adequate and the bathroom was directly opposite. I looked out the little window and could see nothing but fields and fog. It was already sparking off my imagination. I unpacked and put my writing pad on the bedside cabinet. I wondered how much I was going to write while I was there. I wondered if I might go on a writing frenzy and finish the whole book.

So it began. I took a walk once I had settled in, towards the town. I walked past shops with their windows displaying fairy ornaments along with Cornish fudge and other souvenirs. I didn't go in any of them but just wandered through the whole town until I reached the end and the town broke up into residential areas. It was a small picturesque place with some really old buildings and more than a few pubs and restaurants. That suited me fine as I was going to be there for seven nights. There were quite a few tourists about but it wasn't overly busy and on the one road that led into town from where I was staying I had not seen a soul.

If I had gone in a different direction, I would have come to the coast. I had glimpsed the sea briefly when the taxi dropped off the first couple and I knew then that I would be spending quite some time walking the coastline. First things first though, I wanted a beer and some food.

I don't know what people thought of me, eating and drinking alone. They might have thought I was strange, and it was only at those meal times that I felt quite lonely. I sat on my own surrounded by couples and old people in big groups. There were very few children around. ...But I went out for a meal most nights trying out different restaurants each time and then I would buy some alcohol and go back to my room. I would drink, listen to music and write some notes for the novel, although I wrote very little. The holiday was working though. My story was coming to me and the locations and situations came each day and were stored in my head.

In the daytime I put on my stereo and took my bag with me, that had my writing pad and camera in it, and set off on a hike. I walked along the coastal paths looking down at the steep drop and the jagged rocks that tore into the sea. The water thrashed and foamed white below me and I thought, "Just one step and I could be gone". I thought that a lot while I walked from those known places to somewhere new. Sometimes the cliffs were huge and high and I imagined my body falling down and smashing on the rocks. I felt vertigo but I challenged it and kept looking down letting my imagination kill me over and over. That wasn't really how I wanted to go, it scared the hell out of me, but I could not keep thinking of it. Before I got to Cornwall I had been thinking of perhaps taking another overdose while I was there. That way it would be the owners of the bed and breakfast that would find my body and they would have to deal with it rather than my family having to. Sometimes I think the only thing that stopped me was the uncertainty. I didn't want to survive again.

I wore little make up while I was there and although I hated looking in the mirror I never had that awful panic attack that kept me prisoner. I was able to get out of the room each day, and each day I would go somewhere new and seldom saw another human being until I got back. I found a wood and went in there and took photos of huge trees and in there I found a little hexagonal building, like a turret with an open door way and a little square window. I had no idea what it was but I knew I could use it in my book and I took a number of photographs of it. I remembered how in that wood it seemed like it was raining with the sound of dripping leaves all around me. However, it was old rain and new mist, and when I got back out of the wood the rain magically stopped.

I wrote about the mist quite a lot. In the mist you could imagine all sorts of things. It would hang over the sea and the wet mossy fields and you would walk towards it but never reach it. There could be little people living in that fog, little vicious people and then one day I was sure that I had found the home of the piskies. It was a beautiful green glen with a pure stream running through it. I followed the stream to the music of Tori Amos and when I reached the waterfall, crashing through the rocks and falling to the pool below I was suddenly not alone but had joined three hippies who stood in the cold water practicing tai chi.

It was a good experience on the whole. I spent the whole time alone and did not talk to anyone for days. I spoke to myself occasionally, I spoke to the waitresses when I ordered my food, but I chatted to no one. It was just what I wanted and just what I needed. I think that going there, living through that strange experience and fuelling the imagination needed to write my next novel, kept me alive for a whole year. For that's how long it took to write 'Dark Little Secrets' and, although I wanted to badly, I could not go until it was finished.

It was hard to not try killing myself again. Everything in my life was the same and I thought about doing it everyday. I was using drink and cutting myself as a way to keep myself safe, a contradiction in terms. One of the guys at work said, "What have you done to your arms you look like one of those self harming people". It was so far from their world that they didn't even consider that perhaps I was.

I had a new tattoo, the words 'I know it's over' written in flowing script around my bat tattoo. There were many reasons for it. For one, it's a Smiths song, a song that's lyrics sing about loneliness and how the 'soil is falling over my head'. That song had become the soundtrack to my misery and I needed to tell the world what I'd been through. It also meant that my life is over, my old life, perhaps even my new life. I wasn't sure if it was a positive or a negative. I don't even know why I wanted it done so badly; it just begged me to do it and I succumbed. I guess it's the one tattoo that really shows my mental health. If I were sane I probably wouldn't have had it done.

I was trying to live, trying to move forwards but I was never good at putting my old life behind me. I was still in contact with Carey and with Andie, but I tried not to cling to them or see them. Carey moved away from the area although she still e-mailed me and even phoned me occasionally. Everyone told me I should tell her where to go but I couldn't do it. That is a weakness of mine. I don't see the harm that people are doing and I'm not strong enough to say, "You are harmful - please piss off". I had people around me that sucked up any happiness I had and spat it out, but I was learning, slowly. I was learning to get over these people and have a new life.

I saw my psychologist regularly despite the lack of faith I had in therapy. I just wanted them to give me a miracle drug to take it all away. I know that the therapist was finding it hard to deal with me, as I was so pessimistic that I did not welcome any changes. I refused to stop drinking despite the fact that it often led to me cutting. I refused to try and change my train of thoughts from negative into positive. Because I did not change, I felt that I was keeping myself safe from some perceived threat and denied the possibility of improvement. Yet I went each week and I watched her pull her hair out trying to sort me out. She tried to make me focus my coping strategies on my love of music and writing rather than alcohol and razor blades. I found it all laughably impotent, but was this not normal? Weren't all depressives pessimistic and scared of change? Perhaps not.

That summer I had a short relationship that I regret despite how good it probably was for me. I was not well enough for a relationship. I was still thinking that I wanted to be like Morrissey - living alone and staying celibate. I met up with a girl that used to be in the crowd of friends I had when I was younger. We chatted all night at a club, chatting about shit that had happened to us. We spent a good hour or so discussing how unimportant sex was and then began a relationship that had me tackling constantly with that physical demon. Sex, it seemed, was important to her after all and I was still unsure about the whole thing. To me, my sexuality did not define who I was, it just did not matter, but you can't be with someone and stay like that. It only lasted for a couple of months and it only lasted that long because she made me feel so much better about myself. That, I learnt, is not a reason to be with anyone. I led the poor girl on and she said she loved me but I didn't love her. That was a strange thing for me, having to be the one that ended it all. It feels almost as bad as being dumped.

...But my reasons were true. I was really unwell. Cutting myself, drinking and wanting to die was becoming a way of life and I was stuck in the rut. I couldn't think of anything that would make things better for me. I hated my job, I hated myself, I hated people and I hated the world. I had hang ups about everything and my therapy was not touching the sides. I told her that it wasn't helping and we decided to stop it. I still saw my social worker though and I told him all the horrible thoughts I was keeping inside. I also saw a new psychiatrist every three months and when I first saw the new doctor he chose to increase my antidepressants and added a new medication. He prescribed me Olanzapine that he said could help with the fixation I had about my skin. I was willing to try anything. It was just getting worse and worse.

I bought some Sudacream and covered my nose with it each night hoping that new skin would grow. It said it was skin-healing cream so surely it would help. It made my nose look white and seemed that it might work but it never did. I remember that winter and it was the worst I had ever been. I knew that the cold made my nose look more red than normal and I was having a nightmare each day getting it into some condition where I could be seen. It snowed one day so heavily that they let everyone go home from work early. I only lived up the road so I walked back to my house. I was so glad to get home and I ran upstairs and washed my face in warm water. The white snow outside was making the world too bright and in the daylight I looked the worst. I cried when I looked at my bare skin. I covered my face in the Sudacream and went to bed to sob myself to sleep.

The Olanzapine wasn't working. The doctor told me that it was used to treat schizophrenia but that I definitely did not have that. He said it also helps people who are experiencing bad phobias and having disturbing thoughts. It is an anti-psychotic also called Zyprexa. The first thing I did was to look up whether it could be fatal in an overdose. I looked it up on the internet and it didn't sound good. It never does. They were not fatal they just mess you up for a while. I wasn't going to use them, but I kept taking them in the hope that they would kick in to action at some stage.

I didn't know what I wanted out of life anymore. The only thing I knew I wanted was success with my writing but sometimes that just seemed over optimistic. I was also at a loss with how to get over this whole skin thing. I looked up plastic surgery on the internet and wondered whether I should get a chemical peel. I went to a hypnotherapist and told him that I was depressed, skating over the skin problem by saying I simply had 'phobias' and he tried to put me under. It didn't work but it cost me forty quid. I could have done what he did, speaking low and gentle and telling me to imagine my problems as a big black cloud. My problems were already a black cloud and they smothered me. I could have opened my eyes at any point yet I kept them closed hoping that I would suddenly be on that other plane and my phobia would be washed magically away. It wasn't.

I wished that I could be simply depressed, for the depression on its own was bad enough and people noticed. I didn't realise how glaringly obvious it was but then I would hear it back from someone else. Like when I went to the natural history museum with my sister and the kids. I had not been able to sort my skin out and I only managed to leave the house because I didn't want to let them down. I felt suicidal all day, everything made me think of death and how I might just do it as soon as I was home. I was planning it while we walked through the dinosaurs, thinking that I might try slitting my wrists again. I didn't want people to look at me so I was keeping my head down the whole time. I didn't think my sister had noticed but they told my mother and then she told me. "Jane says you were very bad on Saturday, you hardly even spoke." My cover was blown.

There were other times when I knew it was obvious and there was no getting round it. Like when I was sitting at my sister's house eating a dinner they had cooked me and I suddenly started crying uncontrollably, blubbering over my dinner and frightening the kids.

"What's wrong with Uncle Steve mummy?"

What could she say? She said that I had a 'poor poor', a euphemism for 'he is fucked in the head.'

I was crying a lot around that time, any little thing would choke me up. I cried myself to sleep most nights; I cried watching 'Buffy'. I was the worst I had been for ages yet I had not attempted to kill myself for months. I had nothing actually wrong in my life to tip me over the edge. I was just waiting for a reason, whether I was waiting for my own good or for the good of others wasn't clear. If I were to just do it, it would have been a major shock to the family and that would be hard for them. However, if I could prove that there was a build up; if something went wrong in my life that was an obvious trigger perhaps they could come to terms with it, but what could possibly happen in my life? I had no life and that was the main problem. I hid away from the world; I refused to go out; I had no friends. Michael had left his job and I never saw him anymore. I sat in front of my computer writing my novel and going online to see if I had any messages. I never did.

Sometimes I thought that the only reason I was living was that I was waiting to meet 'the one'. I wondered if

I could survive long enough to find her. I had a few dates, which didn't go too well. I was ill and had pain in my face and in my words. I was so nervous when I met one girl that I freaked out about it all day at work, going to the bathroom over and over to see if my face had improved. Then, when I got to the pub I was a gibbering wreck and smoked a whole box of cigarettes telling this complete stranger things that really weren't attractive. I must have come across as a total freak.

I made friends with a South African girl who started to work for Oaklands called Phoebe, and was disappointed when I found out she had a boyfriend. We remained friends and she forced me to get out of the house occasionally. I told her everything in the end and we spent a lot of time talking about how shit life was. She didn't help me to feel any less miserable though. She probably made things worse. I liked her a little too much. We were 'just friends' but while I was going out with her I couldn't meet anyone else. I guess that suited me. I guess I wasn't really ready to meet anyone. A friend was about all I could cope with at that time, so a friend was what I got.

...But if I wasn't looking for a girlfriend to improve my existence then what was I living for? I certainly wasn't living for the life that I had, more the life I thought I might get in the future, but when anyone spoke of the future I just laughed inwardly thinking, "I have no future, I am going to kill myself". Someone at work would talk about a new job that we would have to do in a few weeks time and I just thought "Well I won't be here so it doesn't bother me." I felt sorry that it was true but I knew myself well enough; I knew I had it in me to take my own life and I knew that I would try it again. Planning anything other than my own death was pointless.

'Dear diary,

I am sad and pathetic. I am looking for a way to live yet I just think about ways to die. I think about letting myself in to the tower blocks in Stevenage and jumping out one of the windows. I wonder how secure the entrance doors are and whether the windows fully open. I have never heard of anyone jumping from there but you would certainly die if you did. Can it be true that there has never been a depressive living there? If I lived there I would jump out the window within a week. Or there is the hospital, if I could get to the top of that and jump then that would kill me. I guess I'm too scared to do it that way. I have been thinking of some other ideas and I'm going to do something about it for good.

I find living, close to unbearable. Everything I used to enjoy means nothing now. My writing, my house, my rabbit, my music, it just is not enough. That's what being depressed does to me. I think that finding 'the one' would make things right but that's just pathetic. I shouldn't put so much faith in another person. I wish I wasn't like this. I wish that I could be happy with myself, alone, but it is the times that I am alone and my life is stagnant, that I see no point in any of it. I am obviously better when my life is going well, but I am also happier when my life is going badly, it's the nothingness I can't cope with. So I look for 'the one' and when I think I have found her I get excited and then get terribly disappointed when I discover I am wrong. I suppose I can't expect someone else to give me happiness, but after failing to find it for myself for all these years that is the only hope I have left.

My problem is the way I think and I don't know how to change that. I am only human, and a weak one at that. I'm just so desperate to be happy and I don't see it happening.'

As the spring brought forth life, plans formulated for my death. I had an idea. I went to see my doctor and I told him I could not sleep. This was not true. Although insomnia was a symptom of depression I never had a problem with sleeping. …But there I was looking my doctor in the eye and lying so that he would give me sleeping pills that I could take to kill myself with.

"It's not really advisable for me to prescribe sleeping pills to someone that has had a history of suicide attempts but of course it is not going to help your mental state to suffer insomnia."

Damn he suspected didn't he? Just give me the bloody pills I don't ask for much.

"I will give you a small amount of pills for now and see how you get on. Ok?"

I nodded and I took the script.

"Thank you doctor."

Twelve pills. Could twelve be enough? Could taking the sleeping pills mixed with my other medication be fatal?

I believe quite categorically that I am a suicide junkie. I have it stuck in my head that I am supposed to kill myself and after long periods where nothing much is happening to sway me, the thought of it just gets too much to bear. Too much time had gone past since the last attempt, I was getting the cravings again. If I were supposed to die from suicide then I would have to get on and try again. I certainly didn't want this life. Going to work all day, sitting in an office with my boss hiding from everything, e-mailing Phoebe about how crap our jobs were and what music I was listening to at the time. We spent a lot of time together that summer but she didn't know what was going on in my head, no one knew.

'Dear diary,

I am so close to death that I can hardly breathe. I go to work and I hide somewhere because I just can't do it. I know me; I know how serious this is. This is leading up to something big. I don't know when the final decision will come but I was close tonight. I look disgusting, which shouldn't be such a big deal but it is. I can't bear to be seen and I just want to hide my face away from everyone. I can't bear the pain of rejections, in all aspects of my life, just being told that I am not good enough. These things don't fade away; they just pile up. I can't bear the pain I am going through everyday and I don't enjoy anything anymore; I can't remember the last time I did. I tried to watch a movie tonight and I cried four times before it finished - and then I cried some more later. I am so fragile.

I didn't drink tonight - the first night I have been sober all week. Maybe that's why I can't cope right now. I am not fit for this world - I think I need to die and start again. I'm a mess. I think I will try to get my novel finished real soon and then give myself the dignity of an early death. I can't tell anyone how I am feeling, not even my social worker, because he will just ask me to give him the pills so that I don't take them all at once - he has done that before - but I don't want him to save me this time, this time I truly want it to be the last time, this time I want it to work. I don't really want to die, not really, but I don't want to live either. So what are my options? Crawl back up into the womb and pray to never be born?

Suicide is always dancing behind my eyes yet no one sees it. No one knows how many tears I have cried tonight. No one knows how they hurt me with their smiles and with their flippant comments. No one knows how little things can affect me. My sister is going on holiday soon and I know what I am going to do...'

It was August and my sister and her whole family went abroad on holiday leaving me in charge of the cat. They gave me keys to the house so that I could let myself in to give him food. I rode to the house every lunch break and called him, stroked him a little and gave him his biscuits. I was sweating by this time as it was so hot and I had ridden so fast. I tried to cool down a little before riding back to work. I didn't care about having any lunch; I wasn't eating much at the time.

My sister had been ill for years and she had a huge stock of tablets in one of the cupboards, so I looked for them. I opened the pantry and searched there. I looked in the plate cupboard and where she kept the glasses and finally I opened the correct one and a few white paper bags fell out onto the worktop. She really did have a lot of medication in there, so much that it was falling out. She had bottles, white boxes and pharmacy bags. I took a bottle out trying to see what the tablets were without disturbing anything. I obviously didn't want my sister to know that I had been snooping around in her cupboards. I didn't know what the pills were, but I thought I knew one thing - she took Amitriptyline and as far as I knew they were sleeping pills. Searching in some of the bags I found that she had about five boxes of that particular tablet. She wouldn't miss a single box would she?

I took a whole box of them and put it in my bag, and then I put everything back as I had found it. I felt guilty for stealing something from my sister but she didn't have to pay for her prescriptions so I didn't think it was so bad. She need never know and I would never know if it hurt her because I wasn't planning to live much longer.

I believed with all my intelligence that I had got enough pills to kill myself with this time. I had the sleeping pills that the doctor gave me and now I had these as well. This was the first time that I truly believed that I had no chance of survival. It is a strange feeling knowing that you are going to be dead soon. Everything just goes on as normal yet you feel far from normal. I went back to work and did my job yet I knew that it was all pointless. I didn't care about the things that were happening there and I was glad that I would not see these people again. I left on that Friday and I went into hiding.

I bought a bottle of vodka and went home. I locked my door, drew my curtains and poured myself a drink. Then I went to the bathroom. I covered the window with a towel and washed the make up and the world from my face. I looked awful as always. I wasn't planning to go anywhere for the whole weekend though, time for my face to heal, time to think about what I was going to do, to get used to the idea that I was soon going to die. I was in no rush, it would happen in time.   I popped all the pills out of their blister packets and dropped them into a glass beside my bed. My ticket out of this life, my final escape. I could be happy now, knowing that I didn't have to try and be happy anymore. I could rest now, never again would I have to put on a face. Never again would I have to spend a day at work hating everything and everyone and listening to their foul language. Stephen Westwood was going to be one of those people that had committed suicide.

'Dear diary,

209

I have spent the entire weekend locked away - I haven't seen a soul. I'm too ugly to be seen. It took me an hour in front of the mirror this morning so that I could go to the shop to buy more vodka. I have been drinking all day, writing and staring at the tablets in a glass on my bedside cabinet, scribbling the last words I will ever write and battling my desire to die. I am not going back to work ever again, I text in sick today but made it obvious that it was mental. I don't care anymore. I don't care who knows.

It would be easier to just die tonight; I don't really know what I am holding off for. I have finished my novel but I need to type up the last chapters - I'm not going to die until I have done that. …But once that is done will I think of some other excuse? I am scared, but I will do it. I know I will do it.

I've been feeling kind of numb all weekend. Then I broke down. I'm in tears right now, real tears; at least I know that I am not completely vacant to what is happening to me. I wrote on the forums again and people have replied but words aren't going to change anything now. Every little thing hurts so badly. I can't stop thinking about one sick comment made by someone at work and can't stop thinking that I don't want to share the world with these people. The fact that it hurts me so bad just proves how pitifully sensitive I am. I am too fragile to be here. I am not going to be living much longer and I really don't care.'

I spent the next two days typing up the last of 'Dark Little Secrets' as if it was the only important thing I had left. I wanted to put my affairs in order. I updated my funeral requests that I had at the start of my diary and I printed them out. I wrote a will of sorts and wrote asking that my family try to get my work published for me, but I would not have to deal with the rejections this time. I drank vodka and orange from the moment I woke until the time I went to bed. I slept in my clothes and did not wash or bath. Nothing mattered because I would soon be gone. I was having a break down. My mind was evil and twisted making me pace the house and talk to myself.

"You are pathetic, why don't you just do it now?"

I lay in bed hardly daring to get up to face yet another day, all those hours alone with myself; I didn't know if I could cope. I lay there staring at the glass with the tablets in and I kept daring myself to pick it up and to swallow them down. That was all it would take, a moment of courage, a moment of utter hopelessness and I could be free. I lay for hours scared of looking at myself again. There was a massive cut on my face where I had stuck my own fingernails into my skin. It looked disgusting. I looked at myself lying there with the shard of glass beside the bed and I threw it down in despair at my own ugliness. Tonight, I thought, tonight I will do it.

For all this time I had been utterly secluded. No one knocked at my door. The phone did not ring. No one knew or cared what was happening to me. I texted work each day to say that I was still ill. I don't know why I even bothered doing that. I had no job now.

I finished typing up my novel, saved it on floppy disk twice, and labelled them up. Then I set to writing something that would be my suicide note, a piece of prose to explain it to my family, to make them realise that I had no choice, to make them feel happy for me that I had escaped this hell.

'For frequent tears have run the colours from my life (Elizabeth Browning 1850)

He wanted to give them all something, something to remember him by, but he hadn't much to give. Tens of CDs loved by him but that would never be as loved by others. Video films collecting dust, bought on the off chance that he might, one day, have the energy to sit still and watch one. Films that spoke to him, were part of him, but in real terms were just plastic and ribbon.

If he had money he would divide it and give it to those he loved, but he had always lived hand to mouth. Money in his hand became cider in his mouth. His bank account was in minus figures because it was still six days before payday.

He felt sad, writing out what should go to whom because he knew that they would read it. He knew that when they read it he would be gone. The things in his house would still be there. The clock on his wall would still be ticking. His computer would be there waiting for him to type his password, but he would see none of it again. It made him sad that this was his life.

He knew that no one would understand. No one knew how much pain he was in. No one knew how many tears he cried alone. No one could possibly know how awful it was to be Stephen. To them he had lots of nice things. To them he was a kind, good looking young man. ...But if only they were to spend a day inside his head they would run out screaming.

His kindness was a curse, which made all the harmful acts in the world intolerable. He couldn't watch the news or read the papers. Those things would enter his mind and stay there - one more happy cell destroyed, and people would tell him of their day, yet just one little thing they might say could destroy him. If they had been treated badly, if they had experienced even a moment of pain it would hurt him forever.

...And good looks? If only he didn't expect to look good perhaps the pressure wouldn't turn to obsession. His face mocked him, changing like the tides and never settled. So he could not settle. He was always on show and he always wanted to hide.

He didn't really expect them to understand. He knew that they would never really know 'why'. He only wished that they would forgive him and that they would wish him peace. For it wasn't easy for him, nothing ever was. He didn't want to do this to them, to give them pain, to make them question. It was no ones fault. He had spent years contemplating and it always came back to this. He would try to live but he was always dancing with suicide, and now she was leading.

Five days of solitude. Five days he kept himself hidden, waiting for a sign, but the signs were all there. Every evening the alcohol would allow the tears to flow again and he would sleep, but he would wake in the same place he had left the night before. Nothing was changing. Why was he waiting?

His life had been flashing slowly and painfully in the eye of his mind. Things he had not thought about in years were coming back to see him off. He remembered every happy moment and it hurt him. He remembered every hurtful moment and it broke him. He thought of everyone he had ever loved, he thought of every heartache, and his heart still ached. Nothing was lost. Everything was building up and it could get no further. Every memory, etched in stone, and those stones now piled up high. Now that pile was crumbling down over his head.

He had so much love for everyone but could find none for himself.

It was over. It was time he gave himself what he needed. He had to do this. He could see no way back. He could not imagine living... it was too late to start. If only he didn't have to die.

He was never comfortable being human, perhaps he would make a better angel.'

I took a new web cam picture of myself and put it on the top of the page. I wanted to see if you could see suicide behind my eyes, wanted to see if I looked different. I looked very sad and there was no spark to my eyes. I printed the whole thing out and laid it down on my sofa along with the will and my funeral details. Whoever found me would find them and they would know why I did it and what I wanted to happen now I was gone. I had no remorse. I felt no guilt. This wasn't even a choice anymore, if it ever had been, I had to kill myself; there was no way I was getting back from this.

I decided that I would do it that night. I had run out of vodka so I went to get some more. I didn't even look at myself in the mirror, I just left the house, the first time I had done that in years, but I didn't care now. What did it matter what the shopkeepers thought of me? Buying vodka again, the third bottle I had bought in so many days. If they thought I was ugly then perhaps they would understand why I was drinking so much. They would be the last people to see me alive.

I rode there and back in a matter of minutes and rushed back into the house before anyone could see me. I started the bottle straight away, pouring about four shots into the glass and topping it up with orange juice. I was treating myself by drinking vodka, my usual cider wasn't the last drink I ever wanted to have and money was no object, as you can't take it with you.

I passed the next few hours in my living room, sitting on my sofa and trying not to think about anything that might set a seed of doubt in my mind. I didn't want to talk myself out of it. I had promised myself that this was it and it was going to be it. I wasn't scared. I was resigned to it. I sat and watched 'Girl Interrupted' that I had on video wondering if it would have been better for me to go to a mental institute like the characters in the film. Winona Ryder's character took a whole bottle of Aspirin and chased it with a bottle of vodka; she said she 'had a headache' and she was taken in to the ward. I was crazier than she was and here I was planning to die in my house all alone and no one even cared enough to knock at the door. Perhaps I was going to take all these pills because I 'needed the sleep'. I was looking forward to the rest. I had no doubts.

I was waiting for the evening before I did anything. I wanted to be drunk and I wanted to be sleepy, then I would not feel fear and could just close my eyes for the last final time. I went upstairs to begin the end, taking my vodka with me. I put on suicide tape one and lay down on my bed with my head propped up on the pillow staring at the glass with the pills in it. They were mocking me for my hesitation but I was merely biding my time, savouring my last few moments. I looked around my room wondering if I would miss anything; I decided that I wouldn't. As the cathartic songs played, I thought about how this would be the last time I ever heard them, but I did not rewind a single one to play it again. It was ok that this was it; I was ready.

I had already decided how I was going to take the pills. They were waiting there in a glass and I figured that I could fill the glass with water and take it all down together. It would be easier to do that than popping them one after the other. If I just popped them one after the other I might lose my nerve before I had taken enough to see me off. For although I really wanted this, I really wanted to die, it still took guts to go through with a suicide attempt. It was against human nature to harm ones self and I had to go against the survival instinct that even I had to a certain degree. I didn't have much of it though, my urge to die was stronger, and so I picked up the glass and sat looking down at the pills getting ready to swallow the whole lot.

I got up from the bed with the glass in my hand and went down stairs with it. I went in to my kitchen and put the glass under the tap, filling it half full with water. Then I went back upstairs.

I looked at myself in the full-length mirror in my room, standing there with the poison glass in my hand, a scene of suicide captured but not saved. I wished that I could take a photograph of that image, a poignant arty shot of a man ready to send himself to death. I sat on my bed and stared into the liquid, and then I did it, I took a swig.

The pills did not roll down my throat as I expected and the water tasted of acid; I was very nearly sick when I tasted it. I moved the glass away from my mouth and stared at it, washing the inside of my mouth with my tongue. The pills were dissolving in the water. A moment's courage, a moment of total abandon, and I took the whole glass down.

I recoiled from the taste and put the glass heavily down on the bedside cabinet. It was empty now except for some mushy white stuff stuck to the bottom. I wondered how many of the pills I had actually digested, the taste still clinging to my mouth and making me feel ill, but it was done. I had not had a choice in the end had I? It was what I was destined to do and now it was done and I could lie down and let death take me.

I drank some vodka and orange but my mouth just tasted foul now and the vodka didn't help. I took off my clothes and put on a pair of pyjama bottoms and a t-shirt, and then I crawled in to bed. The pills were not having any affect on me but I knew they would. I had taken a hell of a lot of sleeping pills and now I would go to sleep.

The music came to an end, the tape player made some noises and then the next tape started to play on its own. I listened to each song, each one carefully chosen to make me feel at ease during my final minutes stuck on this drab planet. I listened and I lay and sleep came to take me away.

There is a vague recollection of people calling my name. I heard it as though it were in my head, voices and banging, and banging and voices, and then nothing. My mind swam without thought; I could not place the sounds. They didn't mean anything.

I awoke to a banging on my door and I sat upright suddenly realising what the sound meant. My head rolled and fell forwards, my eyesight catching up moments later. My mind was still asleep, I had no thoughts just an instinct that the knocking needed my attention.

"Steve?" It was my mother's voice. I knew that voice and I knew I needed her but I didn't know why.

I tried to get up by swinging my legs over the side of the bed but the whole movement blacked out my brain and my eyes blurred. It took a few seconds for my physical body and my mind to attune themselves and give me some idea what was going on. Why did I feel so numb and why couldn't I focus?

I remembered and I looked at the glass beside the bed. I had failed again and my mother was knocking at the door and, shit it was my sister's birthday, and here I was trying to regain control of myself after another damn suicide attempt. I was so selfish I couldn't bear to be in my own company. How could I have done this and why hadn't it worked? I was never supposed to see this day.

I stood up on numb matchstick legs and staggered out the bedroom and onto the landing. The door banged again. "Don't leave yet I'm coming..." I needed her help now didn't I? Now I was alive.

I went downstairs, tightly gripping the wooden banister with my hands while leaning my back on the wall. I could not see straight, everything looked different and if I concentrated too much on what I could see I lost control of what I was doing. Focus, left leg, right leg...

I was at the door and I fumbled with the lock and then, the door was open and my mother was there looking all lost and depressed.

"Steve?"

I didn't know what I must have looked like. I tried to speak but my voice got stuck in my throat. I went back into the house and she followed me. I sat on the bottom stair with my head in my hands.

"What's the matter?"

I thought it was obvious, but she didn't know what I knew and she didn't know how awful I felt. My eyes tried to focus on her standing in the doorway.

"I took an overdose."

"No, God Stephen why?" She came into the living room and I stayed where I was my whole head buzzing and my eyes spinning as if I had just downed two bottles of vodka. I felt sick. I could almost taste those pills on my tongue and all I kept thinking was how it was my sister's birthday and I had got a present for her, but now I had done this and she would be upset all day.

"I look disgusting," I said, my voice slurring and my tongue feeling heavy in my mouth. "My face is full of puss."

"I knew something was wrong because you missed your sister's birthday." My mother sounded completely bewildered, like a child.

"Today is Jane's birthday."

"No it was yesterday and she was waiting to hear from you, but you didn't call or contact her at all."

"What day is it?"

"It's Friday."

...And that's when my mind kicked in to gear. I was horrified at what I realised in that moment.

"I slept through a whole day."

The Saviour

I spent the rest of the day at the hospital. My mother called for an ambulance saying that she could not handle this and that she would be along to the hospital later. I was to be alone, just like always. I didn't know it at the time but my mother spent a good hour or so telling my entire family that, "Steve has done it again" and then she went to my place of work and told my boss. Apparently, my boss had come to my house and having been unable to get my attention, had called my mother. She didn't want me to get sacked for having so much time away and I guess she really believed that telling him was a good thing. By that time the whole work force probably knew. I later discovered that my boss's promise to only tell the people that he had to tell was open to interpretation.

The paramedics wanted to know what I had taken so my mother looked through my bins to see if the pill boxes were in there. She pulled out all the drafts of my suicide note - all the copies I wasn't happy with and I felt stupid that I hadn't just burnt them. Then she found what she was looking for.

"Amitriptyline." She told them.

"Ok thank you."

"How did you get them?" My mother was asking but everything was just a tinny noise in my head. I couldn't concentrate on moving my legs and listening to her at the same time. I mumbled a response and even I don't know what I was trying to say.

I don't know what time I got to the hospital or what they did when I was there except I remember sitting on a wheel chair in the corridor waiting for the psychiatrist to come and evaluate me. I sat there staring at the floor and at my stupid black pyjama bottoms and I felt underdressed and on show. By now my family had come. My mother, my father and my sister were there, spending their evening waiting with me to see if I was a complete loony and needed to be locked away.

Earlier I had been in the A and E cubicle and I was waiting on my own and out of the corner of my eye I saw something and turned quickly around. There, standing behind the bed was a little girl holding a bunch of red flowers. It wasn't right, she shouldn't have been there, and then she wasn't. I saw her for only a split second as I turned and then she was gone. I knew that I was hallucinating, but she was so real. I got to wonder if this close run in with death had attuned my senses to the other side. Perhaps that little girl had died in this hospital and what I saw was her ghost.

Now, in the corridor I stared at the floor because there were so many God damn insects everywhere. I sat watching them, watching every little mark on the floor grow spindly legs and stride around the wheel chair.

"What are you looking at?" My mother asked me.

"Spiders," I said without looking away from the floor. "There are insects everywhere. That's one," I said, pointing to one of the marks that had come alive. My dad came forwards and he trod on the mark purposely, as if he were squashing a bug.

"That's got it." He said, but as soon as he moved his foot it was back again. I knew that it was the drugs. I had taken acid enough times to know what a hallucination looks like, but I was fascinated by the floor and I just kept on watching. I actually think I was kind of enjoying it. It was keeping me amused for the hours that we waited there. I can't begin to wonder what my family made of all this. I'm sure, especially to my father, this was a very strange time.

It was the middle of the night by the time we got out of the hospital and I was tired despite the fact that I had slept a whole two nights and a day. My mother took me to her house to stay for a while. She had been told that this was a very serious attempt at my life and that I could easily have died. It was a near miracle that my liver had not packed up. With such a lack of self worth it is hard to imagine what this was like for my mother. I tend to think that if I died she, and everyone else, would just get over it and move on, but if it was my son doing this I would be devastated. I can't put myself in their shoes, fearing the worst if I do not answer the phone or my door, trying to watch me to see if there are any warning signs, but it is my life and I have to live it. If I feel that I need to die, then that is what I need to do. I was not happy to be alive again after this; I had wanted it to work.

I spent another week at my mother's house and again I was signed off work for a month. I didn't know how much longer I would get away with having time off like this, but I wasn't at all well. My body felt weak and I was trembling all over. My hands shook like an alcoholic and I was cold and clinging to the radiator. I felt truly frail in body and mind and I didn't know what I was supposed to do now. Why couldn't I just die? Why was it so bloody difficult? I decided then that I would not try an overdose again, but I did not decide to not try anything. If I was going to live, something had to change.

I got it into my head that the house I was living in was suffocating me and keeping me ill. Perhaps there were too many old memories of Carey and of dark days alone, scared and feeling like death. I had tried to kill myself three times in that house and every day was a struggle to survive.

222

Perhaps the light was wrong in that house and that's why I felt that I was so ugly. Perhaps I needed new mirrors in new rooms. Perhaps I needed to start a fresh.

I went in to town and visited all the estate agents looking for a new place. I was hoping to get somewhere cheaper and having extra money would make things better too. I could afford to smoke then, and that was a habit I had formed in recent months. It started with just having one every now and again or a few when I went out, but now I didn't see the point in not smoking one after the other. Smoking myself to death sounded like a very sane proposition.

While down the town I thought of something I could do to begin the new me. I went to the piercing studio and got my lip pierced. It wasn't quite as much of a statement as a tattoo but I felt good once it was done, I felt it was a beginning. I had changed something, something I had control over. Anything I could take control of was a good thing.

I was busy the whole month that I was off work, looking at new flats in Letchworth and Hitchin. I was busy but getting more and more depressed; losing my momentum with each day that came. Soon I would have to go back to work and things would be just as bad as they always were and give me a year or so, and I would be back in hospital being given an antedate for whatever pills I had digested. My idea for a new life was not going according to plan. All the flats I looked at were horrible.

About a week before I had to start work again I found a little studio flat in Hitchin that was a good size and in a fairly good location. I decided to take it. The move happened soon afterwards, my mother helping me along with her neighbour who had a truck and was doing the job for fifty quid. I really thought this was going to help me. I had de-cluttered and sold a load of stuff that I no longer needed. I was taking this austere little place and making it my 'bachelor pad'. I had never had a place that was just mine before and I even got quite excited at the prospect. The excitement did not last long.

For starters, I now had to travel to get to work. No more could I stay in the mirror until eight o'clock. Now I had to leave at a set time and get the train. I guess that did kind of help. I couldn't be late anymore or I would be really late. I got up two hours early for work everyday to allow myself time to panic. It was quite dark in the flat and that meant that I couldn't see my skin as clearly, which although made me extra paranoid, did help me to get to work. I would do my face in the bathroom and then I would stand under the light fitting in the main room with a hand held mirror up against my face. This I would do each morning but I did manage to get to work. Sometimes I would just take the make up and the tweezers with me and as soon as I got in I would go to the toilets, lock myself in and sort out my face properly.

Despite the posters and photographs I put up in the flat it did not feel like home. I wanted to make my surroundings less important but it soon became obvious that my surroundings were important and that what I had done was move to a dingy, cold little place that made everything harder for me. Harder to get to work, harder to see Phoebe, harder to sort out my skin, and the bed was in the same room as the sofa so what incentive was there to sit down when I could just as easily lie in bed?

Every morning the alarm would wake me and I would feel that flood of despair wash over me as I realised I was awake and had to deal with another day. I would lie there comatose not wanting to get up and sort out my face and travel, and then spend all those hours at a job I had no interest in. I would lie there and think about ending it all again. I would lie there and make plans as to when and how I might try to kill myself.

No one at work knew how awful I felt each day. It seemed they were blissfully unaware that I was a complete head case. I did wonder whether the rumour had got round to them though. They were bound to have wondered why I had been off work for another whole month and none of them asked me. It was like it was a taboo subject, which kind of hinted at them knowing everything. They didn't treat me any differently though; I was still one of the boys even though I was always going to be the black sheep. However, being at work was the hardest thing I had to do, and I had to do it five days a week. I felt that if nothing changed, if I had to go to work until I was sixty-five, I would not make old bones. It was that simple, if I couldn't find a way to stop the way I felt about being with other people I would probably try to kill myself again.

Every night I would come home from work and I would buy a pack of cigarettes and some alcohol, then I was prepared for another night in my lonely cold flat. I would get in, open a can of beer or a bottle of cider, smoke a few cigarettes and check my e-mails. Then I would go to bed. Bed was my new addiction. I felt tired constantly and I had nothing to stay awake for. I would wash my face and go to bed, listening to gentle music and fantasizing about a better life. I would lie there and play out scenarios in my head, scenarios of getting my novel published or meeting a nice girl. I didn't ask for much - just to be well enough to function - just to have something to cling to.

I didn't eat. I slept for hours. When it came to the weekend I would stay in bed until late in the afternoon and then I would get up to smoke a little. Sometimes I would just smoke in bed. My mother probably knew I wasn't doing too well. She would phone me and tell me that she would be over in an hour and she would try and get me out of the flat. At least with a little notice I was able to sort my face out before she came. Then she would suggest that we go to the pub for one drink or go for a walk to get some fresh air into my lungs. I went along with her usually, if I didn't look too bad, but this was no life. I actually dreaded the weekend as it meant so much time alone in that grey room, so much time to think bad thoughts and obsess over my looks.

I was still a prisoner of my skin. I shaved in the dark and went straight to bed trying not to touch my face but always picking at it as I lay there. It was as bad as it had been in the old house, lying there with the shard of mirror held up at arms length wishing I looked better. I managed to get to work most days but I was taking all my make up and creams with me so that I could retouch everything in the work toilets. I would go to the toilets a lot, sometimes getting in to a state of extreme panic as I tried to make myself look better within a strict time limit. People must have wondered where I kept disappearing. I worried that the boss would notice.

It didn't seem to matter how much my mother and others said I looked fine I just didn't believe them. There was one instance where Phoebe and I were going to see a band together and I had booked the day off work, so that I had time to get ready before travelling to London. I could never go anywhere like that straight from work; I needed time to sort out my face, style my hair and try on outfits. Phoebe was the girl but I was the one that spent hours in front of the mirror, she would probably go straight there.

Well, I got up fairly early and straight away I put music on and started on the cider. I was looking forward to seeing the band and I had the whole day away from work. It should have been a relaxing day but it was one of the worst days I have ever had. I made the mistake of deciding to sort my face out early so that I didn't have to worry about doing it at the last minute and getting panicky. I looked dreadful. My nose was peeling and I had spots. Never mind, I had time to sort it out. I scrubbed my nose with a sponge, which made it almost glow with redness, and then I rubbed Savlon into it. Then I applied the usual make up, but all the peeling skin was visible and it looked awful; I looked like a freak. I tried to pick the skin off with tweezers and failing that I scrubbed it all off and started a fresh. The music had stopped ages ago but I didn't leave the bathroom. I had to stay until I made myself look human.

I drank the cider hoping it would calm me down but it wasn't making anything better. I just looked like a monster and my heart was racing. I felt sick with nerves. I looked up at the clock; I still had hours before I had to leave. So I started again with my face and I went through the usual ritual yet every time I did it I looked disgusting and I couldn't bear to be seen looking that way. So I started again, and again, and I cried and collapsed on the bathroom floor holding my face in my hands wishing and praying that it would heal.

I spent the entire day in that damn bathroom and was still putting the finishing touches to my last attempt at making up my face, when the time came that I would have to leave in order to catch the train. I didn't want to go, I still felt sick with anxiety and my guts were twisted. I only went because I couldn't let Phoebe down. I went but I hated it. I thought that everyone was looking at me, and it was hot in the venue and I was sweating, losing the make up I had worked so hard on. I got home that night and looked in the mirror expecting to see a vile creature with dreadful skin, the hideous creature I had been all day. I looked in the mirror and, I looked fine. There had been no reason to worry; there was nothing particularly wrong with my face at all. It had all been in my mind.

Moving to Hitchin meant that my mental health team changed. I was to see a new psychiatrist, a new social worker and a new psychologist, but I could still see them in the Letchworth centre so that I could go in my lunch breaks.

My new psychologist was different to the first lady I had seen. This new lady was kind of jolly and said from the very first meeting that she didn't want to talk about what was wrong with me. How the hell could she help if she didn't know about all the bad stuff? ...But I knew exactly what she was doing. She was making me talk about what I liked in life in order to train my brain to think about the positive things rather than the negatives that I always wallowed in. So we spent most of the time talking about my writing, films and books and not once did I get to speak about my hours in bed and in front of the mirror. I could talk about the bad stuff with my social worker though, and I did, laying it all on his shoulders.

The first meeting with my new psychiatrist was very important. He asked me what my main problem was and I told him about my face. I was always unsure whether to tell them about that - it was embarrassing and they couldn't change it could they? ...But I told him. I told him about cutting and about the suicidal urges. That was what was wrong with me - now do something about it, and he did. Not straight away but soon enough he helped me to get off the current antidepressants I was on and prescribed me a new tablet called Clomipramine. This, I was told, should not only help with my depression but could also help relieve my obsessive behaviour as well. I was very hopeful, hoping that this would be the wonder drug that made everything ok. My social worker gave me the prescription that the doctor had made for me, giving me a week's worth of the drug. Then the social worker said "We are only giving you a week at a time at this stage as it can be very dangerous in overdose." My ears pricked up. "Over a week's supply could be fatal."

They shouldn't have told me that. Straight away I was making plans. I thought that perhaps I wouldn't take the pills at all, that I would save them up and take a load at once. It seemed that they were giving me a ticket out of this hell I lived in. I couldn't help but smile. How could they be so stupid as to tell me that?

228

"I have to tell you that because you will need to take responsibility for taking these tablets. The doctor has researched your case and he really believes that they will help you but obviously you have to take them as directed, three at night."

My new social worker loved the sound of his own voice. He would tell me something and then tell me it again in a different way just incase I hadn't grasped what he meant in the first place. He was a nice enough man, I just found it hard to get a word in, and how could he know how I felt unless I told him? It seemed that I had a bunch of problems but he would only listen to the first problem and spend a whole hour speaking about that. However, he was the only person I could talk to.

My psychologist, a big lady that always seemed particularly happy with herself, spoke about my writing with me and gave me a real kick in the butt to do something about it. I invested in sending off samples of my second novel to anyone that might have a vague interest in it. It is quite an expensive venture in paper, ink and stamps but I did it, filled with a little optimism, but a little was better than none.

I looked up my new medication on the internet. Clomipramine - Anfranil. It is a tricylic agent, a serotonin reuptake inhibitor or SSRI. On reading, it said that it was an antidepressant and an anti-obsessive drug. It said that it targets both depression and obsessive-compulsive disorders. It was also a mild sedative. Wow, the doctor might be right; this could possibly be what I needed. If my skin problem was, in fact, all in my mind then perhaps this was a cure. Perhaps this drug would stop me thinking about how I look all the time. Either that or I could take an overdose of it and it would help me that way. I looked up 'clomipramine overdose' and read about what happens to the body. There were lots of long words and phrases I didn't understand but it didn't sound very nice. It did say one thing at the end though - 'could be fatal'.

For months I had not bothered to go on the personals sites, mainly because I didn't feel able to take on a girlfriend. I was a useless friend to Phoebe and to Michael who had made the effort to get back in contact with me. I hardly ever agreed to go out with them or have them round to my place. Most of the time I just felt so miserable that I didn't think I had anything to offer them. Why would anyone want to be with me? I was depressed, a depressive, and surely, I depressed everyone I came in contact with. However, on some nights I would go on the dating sites and look through the profiles. I was still convinced that she was out there somewhere, the 'one'. I looked for her in every possible place.

One night Michael convinced me to go to see a movie with him and Phoebe. It was going to be a good night hanging out with my two friends, that's how I was supposed to feel, but I was dreading it. I didn't have much time to get ready and I panicked as I looked in the mirror. I wasn't going to do this again; I retouched my make up and just hoped that no one would look at me too closely, and then I left.

I wasn't too excited to see the movie, it was some stupid teen horror flick, but it wasn't too important what we were seeing, what was important was the social interaction - getting out of the house for a change, staying out of bed for a little while. ...But social interaction has never been my strongest point. Michael was on one of his extraverted highs, it was quite over powering and there was Phoebe laughing at him. Then there was me unable to join in. I was on one of my lows. I didn't want to be there, I didn't want to have to try and be sociable, but I didn't want them to notice. I watched the movie and I sat in silence and then I went home. I felt really crumby. I hated myself for being such a bore. How could I live with myself when I was this nervous introvert? Why would my friends ever want to see me again? I didn't want to live like this anymore.

I went in to the bathroom fuelled with self-hatred and quickly found a razor blade. I prized out one of the three blades and knelt with my arm over the toilet - then, quite quickly and with some force, I slashed the blade across my inner wrist. The cut was fairly deep just below my hand and started to bleed right away, but this was not going to be another self-harming episode. This was more serious than that. I aimed the blade over the cut I had already made and slashed at it again. I winced with the sharp pain but I wasn't finished. I did it again and again in that same place, cut over cut, the pain making my teeth clench until it became far too sore to cope with and the wound was deep and gaping open. It was bleeding but it was not pumping out, merely running in little red streams down my arm. How much did you have to do to successfully slit your wrists? Why wasn't I strong enough to do it?

I stayed there for some time watching the blood run from the wound and drip into the toilet, but before too long I realised that this had failed and I was going to need stitches. I called my mother and I told her half the truth. I told her I had cut my arm and needed her to give me a lift to the hospital. I did not tell her that this was another suicide bid.

The hospital staff are always so nice despite the reasons I was there. They never told me off for having done it to myself, they were understanding and caring and although I always felt guilty for wasting their time, they never gave me any reason to. They gently cleaned the blood from my arm and cleaned up the wound. It was a large open cut on my wrist; I didn't understand why it had not worked. How far down were my veins?

They did not give me stitches. They gave me staples. They held the wound shut and shot me with a staple gun. It hurt and I wondered if they had chosen to use staples in order to teach me a lesson not to do this sort of thing to myself. I still enjoyed being fussed over. There is part of me that likes people looking after me when I feel so low. Perhaps I should be admitted.

Stapled and bandaged I went home and my mother made plans to see me the next day, being Saturday, and Sunday as well. She didn't want me to be alone.

As weeks went by, things began to change. I started spending less time in bed and less time looking at my face. I would shave in my dark bathroom and go to bed without looking at myself. I figured that if I didn't look, I couldn't get upset and I wouldn't start picking at myself and causing cuts. Then, in the morning I would go through the usual ritual but without the panic. I didn't look too bad; my skin was going through a good patch, but this went on for over a week. So I started to think that perhaps my skin had healed, that it was no longer thin, that I would no longer get face-deforming spots and that my nose would not peel.

I stopped taking the make up and things to work and even while there I looked at myself less. I would use the toilet and take one glance in the mirror as I washed my hands but would not freak out. I would not start rubbing my nose or picking my pimples, I just looked and thought, "Well that's what I look like today". Yes I still wore make up but I wasn't obsessed with it anymore. I didn't spend all day thinking about what I looked like or what other people were thinking about my face. I couldn't believe it but it seemed that the problem with my looks had been all in the mind. The crippling phobia about my skin had all but gone and I realised that I had Clomipramine to thank for that. After I had finally told my doctor my most secret symptoms he was able to diagnose me. He said I had dysmorphobia, which I found out was also called body dysmorphic disorder, or BDD, and in doing that and prescribing the new meds, he had saved my life. Now I knew that my problem was

232

psychological rather than physical I could start to get better. Fifteen years of suffering had all but come to an end. I owe him more thanks than I could ever imagine.

...But I was waiting for it to go wrong again. Every morning I dreaded going into the bathroom in case all the previous problems came back, but it went on for weeks and I began to relax a little. I was free of that one thing that held me back and I wondered if I could start living now. I wondered if my depression would all go away and the new, handsome Stephen could get out into the world and have a life. However, although not having the skin problem was a wondrous relief I was still having suicidal thoughts every day and for every reason. I still had hang ups about the whole human condition. I was still miserable.

I always believed, through my hopeless despair, that I would meet someone through the internet. It seemed obvious that someone was out there somewhere. Someone like-minded, someone better than those trite dating profiles that just wanted to 'have a laugh'. I wanted someone with more than one brain cell, someone that could be serious as well as fun. I wrote in my diary about who would be my perfect partner - someone that was all those things, someone that was a bit of a Goth, someone with big eyes like Christina Ricci. Was I asking too much? Should I be so specific? I would go on the sites every now and again but I would get so disheartened that I would turn the computer off and swear not to look on them again. Then, a week later, I would be back on them. I didn't know if I really wanted a girlfriend, I didn't know if I was well enough, but I realised that I was probably as well as I was ever going to get.

Michael left town to start a new life with his girlfriend and Phoebe went back home; I was alone with only my family as friends. Now was the time to seriously look for a girlfriend. I even said it to one of my work colleagues; I said that I needed to get myself a girlfriend. One afternoon, while not at work (again) I went online, went on to one of the dating sites that I hadn't looked at for a while and logged in.

'You have one new message.'

I had never been sent an e-mail to tell me that I had a message but I had one just the same. I was very excited; this couldn't have come at a better time. I looked at my arms, at the scars and fresh cuts and I wondered if this mystery girl would actually be interested in me if she knew my dark secrets. Perhaps it could have come at a better time after all, it could have come when the cuts had healed, or it could have come ten years ago. I clicked on the 'new message' link. It wasn't a full message it was what the site called an 'ice breaker'. It said 'Did it hurt falling from heaven?' This was a line chosen among others to introduce this girl to me. I was trying to keep calm, as it was early days yet, this girl might be completely wrong for me, she might not be into alternative music or be understanding or have big eyes! My criteria for a girlfriend would be hard to live up to.

I clicked on her profile and there was a girl, a girl I had not seen on the site before, a girl that had the biggest most beautiful blue eyes I had ever seen. I was transfixed to the screen, sitting forwards on my chair and looking at this stranger that I could possibly get to know. I was smiling to myself with sheer excitement. I had been waiting for this, had been waiting for her and here she was. I knew that this was her, but I had to try not to be too excited as this was my life remember, and nothing good ever happens to me.

I read more about her and she sounded very nice, she said people thought she was weird, which was a good sign for me, although there was one problem, a possible big problem, it said that she was soon moving to New Zealand.

Perhaps this wasn't my girl. She looked like my girl, she sounded like my girl but if she were going away I would just be hurting myself if I got involved. I was so sure though, so certain that this girl was going to come into my life. I was so sure and so excited that I paid the thirty pounds it cost to become a full member so that I could send her a message.

'Hello there, thanks for your message it really cheered me up. The site doesn't e-mail me when I get an ice breaker so I had no idea that someone had sent me one. Anyway, from looking at your profile I reckon we might actually be suited. I know what it's like to be seen as 'weird', people often think I'm scary until they get to know me which is pretty funny because it couldn't be much further from the truth. People at work call me 'the lord of darkness'! So what do you do for a living? I'm working for Oaklands at the moment. I'm not really ambitious when it comes to work - I go every day to pay the bills but what I really want to be successful in is writing. I've written two novels and am planning a third. Trying to get published is a nightmare though. My other love is music. I have a wide taste but it's all alternative stuff. What are your tastes? It would be good to hear back from you. Take care. Steve.'

The site wasn't working properly when I went to send the message and I was getting impatient and over excited. I was anxious too. I was getting scared thinking of actually meeting this girl. Could I actually go through with this? I wrote in my diary as I had no one to talk to and a million things going round in my head. I wrote about everything that had happened so far, and my initial feelings.

'...I don't know if the message-sending thing is working, maybe it's just taking a while. I don't know what I hope to achieve e-mailing a girl that is leaving the country soon but I guess I'm just a glutton for punishment. It's just that she looks like everything I have been looking for. She even looks like Christina Ricci with those beautiful huge eyes and black eyeliner. She's really cute. I had to get in contact with her.

Today I had my staples out and I was going to do something like go up to London but I ended up buying a book to read instead. I'm going to sit in the communal garden out back, drink beer and read how a book is supposed to be written hoping it will give me inspiration for my own writing. I have had nothing but rejections for my latest book, perhaps it just is not good enough, perhaps the next one will make my millions.'

The next day, after I had already lost hope that she would actually write back, I had a new message.

'Hi I'm actually really pleased you hit me back as you're pretty much the reason I joined the personals site.' That was a good start and that's why I hadn't seen her profile before... 'I'm surprised we haven't bumped into each other as I lived in Hitchin a while back and have only just moved back to Stevenage after a bad break up. I'm actually more a movie fan than music but I do like a variety of music. I'm really into fifties rock 'n' roll actually but I'll listen to most except rap and r 'n' b and stuff like that.' So she hated the same music that I hated! Having hates in common is probably even more important than liking the same things. She was winning me over quite easily. The rest of her message was just chatting about what she had been up to last weekend, and then at the end of the message she said 'I hope that you'll say hi again and maybe we can even go out for a drink? See you, oh lord of darkness! Ashley'.   And she gave me her mobile number.

I was really excited now, now that I knew her name, now I knew that she was a nice person as well as the fact that she looked exactly like the girl I had been dreaming of. I decided to write back straight away, I wasn't going to act 'cool' or anything, and I just thought that if she was online right then she would get my message and she might write again! I was rushing this along, the tentative e-mailing stage was scary and I wanted to find out more and more about her, and maybe go for this drink she had promised me. However, that very night I had cut myself and now if we did meet for a date I would have to wear long sleeves. That scared me, the thought of having a 'date'. I hadn't been on a date for some time and my history with girls was messed up, but I had a good feeling about this one, I really did.

I sent her a reply and said:

'I think we should probably meet up if you fancy it - maybe this weekend? I'm not the most confident of people but I'll try my best. There's no point me being on a dating site if I'm not prepared to go on a date is there? We could go to Stevenage leisure park and play pool and watch a movie, maybe 'The Day After Tomorrow' as I think that sounds good although it will probably scare the hell out of me - I have a phobia about tidal waves. What movies are you in to? I'm not going to tell you what my favourites are I'll just let you tell me yours then pretend that I agree with you! Anyway - Let me know about Saturday.'

I sounded quite nonchalant and even confident but hey - I could be more confident now couldn't I? Now I didn't have to hide my face away from the world I could arrange a date and actually make it. I still had a million other reasons to be worried but if this was what I wanted then I had to stick my neck out. I gave her my number and she replied after just a few minutes.

'Steve - Hi! I'm still online so I got your message. Huge cheesy grin on my face so it's all good! I can be shy too but I'm also pretty confident so it'll be cool. We can hang out and have fun. As for pool I am the worst player at pool ever. I am really good at getting the white ball in the pocket. Hell, I've even hit the white ball had it bounce over the red then go straight in the pocket! At the time I thought that was awesome but then we lost. ...But yeah it sounds like fun so long as you like winning! Seeing that film would be fine too. I want to see it and am likely to get scared from it too. My favourite movies - wow there's a question but here goes... Labyrinth, Harry Potter (though I prefer the books), Ghostbusters, Rocky Horror Picture Show, Beetlejuice, Edward Scissorhands, anything by Tim Burton actually, Carry on films, Star Wars...God too many to mention. I'm sure you'll mention some and I'll say yeah I love that too. Well I'm free tomorrow night if you are. Take care. Ashley.'

If I should have been playing hard to get about all this I just wasn't. I e-mailed her straight back.

'This is quite exciting but I think we should make the date for Saturday - that way I'll have time to prepare myself'

I was still worried about not being able to make the date. It was a habit I had formed that I thought I needed a few hours to get my face straight even though I was a lot better about it now. I would only have about an hour to prepare if we went on the Friday and that was too much of a worry, but hey! It was nice that she was keen.

'From what I know of you I think we will get on fine. I'm not the best pool player in the world but I enjoy playing it. I think we should do it. I can't believe you said that Labyrinth was your favourite movie... I have one movie poster up in my flat and what is it? It's Labyrinth! I love anything Jim Henson does and I like Tim Burton too. So we have something in common! Anyway - how about Saturday at seven o'clock? I don't drive I'm afraid, I never learnt and I'm scared of cars, so I would be getting the train. Does that sound ok? Let me know. Good night for now. Steve.'

I left her my number. I was going to wait a while and then see if she answered again. I was hoping the fact that I didn't drive wouldn't put her off. I began to worry that it would and that there were so many things that could put her off me, and then she phoned! I am rubbish at phone calls. I fear silences and having nothing to say. It would have been the scariest thing that could happen if she hadn't been so chatty and confident and just really nice to talk to. We spoke for hours, literally about two hours and we got to know more about each other and then chatted as if we already knew each other, as if we were already partners. We spoke of how rubbish work was and how we hated chart music. She told me about her little dogs. We just talked and we laughed, and we started our relationship. She sent me an e-mail later and said at the bottom 'great chatting with you - you can safely say I'm smitten' and I guess I was too.

I think everyone is looking for that special someone really. I think that is what humans are designed to do. I think it was Plato that suggested that we were all one being and then we were split into male and female - two halves - and we spent the rest of our lives looking for the other half. I like that, the whole soul mate theory. I hoped that this was it because the constant searching was hard work. I did not cope well as a single man and my bachelor pad was more like solitary confinement. I pinned all my hopes on Ashley and I believed I had found the one thing that would save my life.

'Dear diary,

I met Ashley yesterday! I was very nervous but I truly believed that everything would be ok, that she would like me. I wore grey jeans, a plain black t-shirt and a black shirt thrown over the top to hide my arms. I had no problem with my skin although I did spend quite some time getting ready. My hair went fine.

I waited around at the bottom of the steps that led from the train station into the leisure park and then I saw someone walking towards me. I didn't know if it was her but she had long black hair and she was coming my way. I felt butterflies in my stomach and nerves took over. As she got nearer I saw that it must be her and she was smiling at me, such a beautiful full-face smile, and it was for me. Her eyes were sparkling, she held her hand out and I took it and we said hi - and I was on a high - I was actually looking forward to something - For the first time in years I had the future on my mind rather than my death. I wanted to have this date, I didn't want to hide, and here was this girl, this special girl, on my arm, liking me, laughing and smiling with me. I wasn't even nervous, not really. She had come at the right time - I was ready for this and I wanted it so badly. Later I was chatting to her in the bar and her eyes kept pulling me in, they were such huge deep pools of blue, I had to shake my head to stop myself from drowning. I liked her already and I just hoped that I wasn't going to fall back down to earth.

I had wanted to give Ashley a present when I met her so I had recorded a tape of mixed songs for her. I wanted to introduce her to some music that I really loved and hoped that she would like some of it too. I gave it to her and she gave me an excited kiss, which took me unawares but injected a boost of confidence through me. She obviously liked me and as I liked her, I felt really quite happy.

In the cinema I kissed her and she didn't' mind. We were sitting on the 'lovers' seats' and it really felt like that - that we were lovers. There was no way this was wrong and I let my guard go completely. I truly believed that she would not hurt me and despite the cliché, it felt like we already knew each other and that I didn't have to hide anything from her. We sat close together as though we were partners for life. She drove me home and in my flat, that dingy place that was once the epitome of my loneliness, I asked her to stay over with me. It was a risk to ask her that, it could have given the complete wrong impression, but I had been without her for so many years I didn't want to be without her again. We slept all night just holding each other. There was no pressure to have sex; we just wanted to sleep in the same bed so that we didn't have to end the date. With her here, my flat seemed much more welcoming and friendly. We ended up in deep conversation and I told her the truth about my scars - she wasn't frightened away - she understood perfectly and admitted that she sometimes did it herself. I knew that my make up would be gone in the morning and that did concern me yet I truly felt that Ashley would not find me ugly. This is the beginning. I can't wait to see her again.'

It was bank holiday and Ashley asked me what I would like to do. I said that I would like to go to the seaside. So that's what we did. It was the best day ever. She came over to my house on Sunday night and we got drunk and watched Labyrinth. Then we went to bed. We did not do anything sexual and I think that was my fault, but it hadn't spoilt anything. I put that aside and thought to myself that we had all the time in the world for that. I did worry about it though. I worried that Ashley might be more experienced than me. Hell, everyone is more experienced than me. I didn't want my sexual hang-ups to spoil the relationship that seemed to be forming. That thorn was in my side but I tried to ignore it and enjoy all the things we did have.

Monday morning we woke up with each other both looking forward to the day ahead. Ashley drove us to Great Yarmouth and we had the best time. We went on some scary rides, we played on the dance mat games, we shot video zombies and we had a few drinks and some seaside food. I wanted to do something exciting to mark this sudden change of fate, so I got my nipple pierced! It hurt. We kissed and held hands all day - I smoked a lot because I was still nervous. I wanted to impress her, but I didn't put on any act. We were both ourselves and I was seriously happy - the happiest I had been in years. If this girl was going to make me as happy as this all the time, I figured I should marry her!

We got back to my house early that evening and we both had baths, then we went to bed and we made love. Every time I have sex it excites me but it scares me. I worry that I'm not going to do it right. It feels like I am losing my virginity all over again. I worry that my incompetence is painfully apparent, yet with Ashley I didn't have sex, I made love, for the first time in my life, and it felt right. I realised that this is what happiness feels like.

The next day Carey phoned me to see how my date went and although I should have just told her to stop being so nosey and to leave me alone, I told her all about it as if Carey was my best friend or something. I didn't have anyone else to tell so I let all my excitement come out and told her everything. She said she was happy for me and said that she had a good feeling about this girl. She said she thought it would last. I don't rate Carey as a fortune-teller but this time I believed that she was right. I certainly hoped so.

Ashley and I did a lot together. We wanted to share experiences and good times. We went to the Cambridge 'Strawberry fair' and I walked hand in hand with her feeling proud to have her with me, happy to be a couple now and to not be alone. I didn't have to be depressed anymore; I didn't have to be lonely. We went to Warwick castle and Woburn safari park. We enjoyed life.

Getting to know a new person is exciting and someone wanting to learn about you is flattering. The first few weeks with Ashley were days and nights of exciting discoveries. We liked similar things, hated similar things, shared views and discussed views. Ashley was intelligent and knowledgeable - she was very mature for her age and was only twenty-one. The fact that I was older than her by some years was fine and Ashley had apparently decided that her next boyfriend should be an older guy. She told me how she had first seen my picture on the site and how she just knew she wanted me.

"I wrote a letter to my guardian angel when I was feeling really low." She told me. "It was about how my ex was not the man I wanted to be with because you are the man I wanted to be with. I didn't know you then but I knew I wanted you. I prayed for you and you are the exact same man that I wrote about."

"Really?" This seemed a little odd to me, but I had done something similar, I had written in my diary about the sort of girl I wanted and here she was. I don't know if all lovers believe this but it does appear to be destiny. It really does seem like magic. It is too perfect to be mere chance. How can two people meet and be so right for each other? There were so many things I didn't like about people in general and Ashley was none of these things. Ashley was everything I had on my wish list and it appeared that I was also the one for her.

This is the letter that Ashley wrote, the letter that was about me...

'Dear Jack,

I know you said I could tell you anything, and lately things have been so bad as you know, and I find myself dreaming of better things. The better thing is a person. I thought I'd tell you who he is. He is my perfect soul...

He has shoulder length hair, straight but with a slight wave and it is either a very light white blonde or a raven black. His eyes must be ice blue, this is not negotiable, and should be startling, with an evil glint. His face should be angular, delicate, yet also he should have strong cheekbones and his nose should be a prominent feature, - perfecting straight but it goes up slightly at the tip. His bottom lip sticks out slightly more than his top. His teeth should be good and strong, but not perfect. His canines should be quite prominent, but not huge fangs, just noticeable. His ears should be a bit elvish and they (well, at least one) should be pierced.

He is slim, but by no means skinny. He shoulders are fairly broad and his waist small. The tops of his arms and his forearms are well pronounced and refined. He has some battle scars on his arms. His hands are masculine, but smooth, not calloused, and he wears his nails quite long and if he decides to paint them, he only uses black or blue. He wears silver jewellery and he has tattoos. His skin is creamy pale and soft, but his arms and back can tan from the sun and leave freckles over his nose. He is angelic, if not elvish in appearance, but when his smile fades he is demonic.

His voice is gentle and soft and he can sing and play drums/guitar/piano. He is poetic and a writer. He can still remember his childhood perspective on things and this magic that comes with being a child. He writes a lot, and perhaps keeps a journal of his thoughts and feelings rather than daily activities. He is experienced with the ways of the heart. He has set opinions on certain issues but would never force them on anyone nor ridicule their opinion should it differ from his. His music taste would be considered alternative, perhaps he's even in a band, but he also appreciates beautiful singing - a woman's voice touches his heart more than a guitar solo.

He would say sweet things often and never forget the small things such as an "I love you" or a compliment. He notices if I am feeling low and comforts me when I cry even if it is because of him or he is angry with me at the time. He doesn't force me to tell him things if I can't, and he keeps a respectful amount of mystery about himself, just enough secrets to remain elusive and tells me enough so I can say I know him well.

He is spontaneous and creative. He decides a sudden trip or holiday on a whim. He turns up at my work place unexpectedly or leaves flowers in my car. He appreciates my affection and does not find it smothering. He feels proud when I stand by him or kiss him in the presence of his friends. He understands that when I tell him I miss him, it is not forcing him to see me, on the contrary it is just an observation of how I feel and that really I am glad we are apart so that we have a chance to miss each other.

He is not a sportsman; he does enjoy swimming or playing crazy golf for example, but as a novelty, - not as a follower of sport or teams. He does not entertain the idea of suffocating crowds of people invading his space, nor of casual sex or betrayal. He has eyes for only one, and he is and always will be faithful.

He dresses casually, in jeans and t-shirts, and trainers (Converse), but he has an artistic flamboyant flair and he likes his gothic clothing, or even pirate, just beautiful clothing that makes peoples heads turn. This, coupled with my own confidence, can enable us to demand that the world bow before us.

He can discuss philosophies of others and of his own; he can speak of death and of dreams. He is not religious but spiritual, but he educated himself on it enough to make a decision. He can be cynical of the generics, a true King of his own court, and I shall be his princess. He is empathic and often things pain him, he has his own agonies yet he still understands mine and why I hurt myself, - perhaps he did it to himself once.

Divided we were lost and floating souls, yet united we are powerful. When together the whole world fades to black and only we exist...He and I versus the World. No on can penetrate our barrier, - they are met with demons and angels if they try.

He is generous, but not suffocating. He will buy me treats but does not lavish and embarrass me. He accepts my independence. He often makes me gifts rather than buys, he writes me poems, stories and songs, draws pictures or perhaps gives me something he found, like a pretty flower, or unusual stone. He appreciates nature; he sees the magic in falling snow and will happily play in it with me. He sees autumn's immense beauty; he loves the colours and the fun of Halloween. He will take my nephews trick or treating with me, and we will answer the door to every mini Frankenstein and vampire that knocks. We drink hot chocolate, eat nuts, treacle tart, and watch horror films and then he holds me tight through the night so that I am not afraid.

He likes summer too; he spends lazy days with me by rivers, with a picnic of strawberries, chocolates and wine. We would spend summer visiting far away exotic countries, enjoying the sights and culture. He enjoys discovering new places that we can dream that only we have ever seen. He will take me to Tintagel and relive the fantasy of Camelot with me with Knights and maidens.

Springtime is his time to dream, and for us to visit castles and forests. We search for fairies, he believes in them you see, and he'd encourage my world of fantasy where we ride a Pegasus, stroke unicorns and spy on sleeping dragons.

He likes to read as well as write, he has similar tastes to me, he loves Harry Potter, and he knows Clive Barker's work. He would probably like Anne Rice too, Vampire Lestat is his favourite.

He is not scientific, but he can and does discuss theories on evolution, time and space. He is a firm believer in all things paranormal and he believes in Guardian angels.

Life with him is a fantasy that I don't wake up from. I want the fairy tale, I want the prince and to be his princess. There will never come a time when it becomes stale and the image of magic fades. I often question myself if maybe he himself is an angel, a dark angel.

He notices the little things in life, and points them out. Like an unusual coloured flower, a ladybug on a leaf that I can catch and ask it to grant my wish, a cute baby rabbit in a field, a bright new moon, the first star at night. He finds these all special. He is kind to animals, and he likes dogs very much, he will love my dogs and we will be a family.

He likes films; he loves Labyrinth especially and anything by Tim Burton. He likes films with a story that can touch your heart, for good or bad, but he does enjoy a horror flick and trashy Hollywood blockbuster.

He is family orientated, he loves his and he will love mine. He would be a great father himself one day, we'd have a daughter and we would show her the hidden magic of the world, she would have a beautiful life.

He likes water, he finds it calming and soothing. He likes to swim, he can even dive and he will teach me and we will swim with dolphins and even sharks! He will show me the wonders of the ocean and we can marvel together at the colours of the marine fish as we sit on the yacht we rented for a holiday in the Caribbean.

He likes the dark, but loves the warm glow from a candle. He uses strawberry scented joss ticks. He lights candles in the bathroom as we share a hot bubble bath and drink sweet wine. He gives massages, sensual ones with warm scented oil. He plays with my hands and strokes my fingers. He can make love to me for hours as we shut the whole world away.

He has a great sense of humour; he can be dry and fairly quick-witted, but never cruel at the expense of someone else (unless we hate them or they're generic sheep - in which case he toys with them like a cat does a mouse). He can be dark humoured and wicked, yet also silly. He finds Lee Evan's funny. He likes The Simpsons and Monty Python.

This is who I'm searching for; he must exist out there somewhere? I know I probably don't deserve him, but please my angel, bring him to me? I will cherish, love and adore him, I promise. Please reveal him to me?'

Well that was crazy, because it was at least ninety percent accurate. It was a description of me, even down to the simple things like the shape of my nose and the scars on my arms. I found myself doubting that it could really be true, but I trusted Ashley entirely and didn't think she would ever lie to me. Had she really written this before she met me? Had she written this when she was with her ex, dreaming of a better life and describing me in her fantasies? Some of it wasn't accurate, but that just made it all the more believable. My hair wasn't long and although I now know from Ashley everything about Clive Barker, I had not yet read any of his books. Some little things were wrong but so many others were right. When I met her that first night, dressed in black with my Converse sneakers on, she must have thought back to that letter and thought that she was dreaming. It is the single weirdest thing I have ever experienced in my life. This is proof that God is not random, that people can be destined to be together. Did I even exist before Ashley conjured me up? I was going to act as though I didn't, as though all the past meant nothing, and now I was Ashley's whole-heartedly.

Despite everything being so perfect it was obvious that misery was there behind the door but both Ashley and I were putting all our weight in to keeping it shut. The world has a way of ruining things though doesn't it? You can't just shut everything out forever. Ashley and I had a few hurdles to jump before we could run the home stretch. Work was one thing. They changed my job, promoted me of sorts, but what it changed to was a spirit crushing, boring, pointless job that I didn't know how to do well. They set up two people to do this job, a job it only really took one person to do, and I was the one that didn't know what he was doing. I hated it - every minute of it. I didn't want to go anymore and those dark clouds started rolling over my Ashley coloured sky. I took days off so that I could be with Ashley and not feel that despair that had come back at full force, for I couldn't see a way out of this. I had to go to work so that I could pay for my flat but I hated it there so much that I would rather stay at home alone if need be. I panicked about going in, not because of my face now but because I couldn't cope with seeing all those people and doing that job.

Ashley hated her job too. We met up a few nights a week and we bitched about life and how the rat race grinds us down. Neither of us were happy in what we were doing and something had to give. I could see this going in the direction of a suicide pact again and I sometimes believed that if I asked Ashley to do it she probably would. She had just got through a bad break up with a guy that stifled her like Carey had done me. She had wanted to run away, and she had chosen New Zealand, thankfully I was enough to change her mind, but to lose a dream, to be told that there is nowhere to run just makes you trapped and miserable. …But truthfully, the only way to run away from your life is to die. We spoke about getting hold of some cyanide and we could keep it by just in case. We both felt like dying, but only if it was together.

The next thing to go wrong was that my flat was no longer available to rent. The owners wanted to move back in. I didn't know what to do; should I suggest to Ashley that we move in together even at this early stage? She was back living with her mum which was not good for her and I hated being alone. I did not ask her right away. We were still enjoying the dating stage of the relationship. We would both get ready before seeing each other, dressing nicely and wearing our best underwear. We watched films together and made love constantly. It seemed a shame to change what was working so well.

One night Ashley and I went out together to the club in Hitchin. We got dressed up in our finest black garb and went there with good spirits. I had been to that club so many times but I had no idea that this night was going to be important, but then it was.

Ashley had been quiet for some time and then she leant over to my ear and spoke. "I don't know if I should be telling you this, and I know you probably don't, but... I love you."

I was taken a back; I really hadn't expected such a declaration. I hadn't really thought about admitting to love at this stage, perhaps it was that my guard was still up a little, perhaps I thought that I should have learned my lesson from Andie, that it wasn't right to declare love in the early stages no matter how deeply you had fallen. However, now Ashley had said it and I wasn't going to let her feel that it was all one sided.

"I do though," I said and I said that I didn't understand why she loved me. I didn't feel worthy of anyone's love but especially the love of this wonderful person. …And the feeling was mutual.

"Then say it, I want to hear you say it."

It wasn't hard for me now, I wanted this to be the start of something really serious and my feelings were obvious.

"I love you Ashley" and we embraced like we had never been kissed.

251

I felt loved by Ashley, and I had never felt that before. I often wondered what it would feel like to be loved, rather than to just love unrequited or twisted in friendship or adoration. Ashley loved me, and she knew me well enough to love me, and I believed her because I felt the same. Ashley was a wonderful girl, an honest, deep and beautiful girl. We enjoyed being together and that was all we wanted. There was nothing else. We didn't want everything else that came with life. We just wanted all our time to be together. It seemed right, then, that we should move in together.

We got a flat in Letchworth so that it would be easier for me to get to work again, though I was strongly considering leaving the job. It had got to the point that I actually thought I would rather kill myself than go there. I hated it so much and it was the main thing keeping me depressed. The other thing keeping me depressed was my stupid mind. The other me in my head was laughing at my relationship with Ashley. It was laughing, mocking and saying how it will all end in tears and that it is only delaying the inevitable. The inevitable being that one day I would just decide to kill myself and I thought that he was probably right. Life with Ashley might be the best life gets but it didn't wipe out those suicidal thoughts. Why? Because nothing life offers is enough for me - it is absolutely no reflection on Ashley at all, she is the best thing that has ever happened to me, but however good life gets it is still life and still, fundamentally, a waste of time. If it is so easy to die why do any of us bother? Life is a struggle and death is freedom. It is only the actual act of killing myself that puts me off doing it. There is no nice way to die.

I told my social worker how I felt and we discussed why I might feel this way, but none of it made sense. Why would I still feel like killing myself when everything was going so well? Why was nothing ever enough for me? Why was it preordained that the way Stephen Westwood was to die was by his own hand? Why was that what I wanted?

The Clomipramine was getting rid of one obsession but the obsession with death was still hanging around me and tempting me away from a life with the girl I loved. She would talk to me about how she and I felt depressed but I couldn't tell her about feeling suicidal - what a kick in the teeth that would be to know that your love wasn't enough to make that person want to live. However, this was me we were talking about - Stephen Westwood the suicide junkie - the failed writer - the warehouse worker - the guy that had wanted to die since he was a kid. You can't break a habit like that easily, and depression had definitely become a habit.

Ashley and I lived together now with our Chihuahua in a fairly good sized flat. We had nice things, we didn't want for much and we were happy together. We never argued we were always touching each other, kissing and telling each other how much we loved them. Ashley would say that I was beautiful, and I needed to hear that, my paranoia still lingering like the smell of smoke, but things were, generally, really good. So what happened? Why wasn't I cured of depression?

One night I was feeling particularly bad and I couldn't hide it. No one has ever been able to see when suicide is burning bright and dark in my eyes, but Ashley knew. She noticed that I was not speaking; she noticed that I had been withdrawn for days and she kept asking me if I was all right. I wasn't all right. I was planning how I might do it, how I might let Ashley go to sleep and how I would stay awake, take all my pills into the living room and swallow them. I had been thinking about it for days and now I had got to the stage where I actually thought I might do it. Then I told her - no I'm not all right, I am having bad thoughts again...I want to kill myself. It was late in the evening when I finally broke down and told her and then the tears came, tears I had been holding on to for days. I cried like a child, sobbing as if the whole world was ending, because for me it nearly was that bad. I was so close to suicide that I could taste its acidic flavour in my mouth. All choice had gone and wanting to die had taken over. I was going to do it if someone didn't stop me and that became Ashley's job.

My social worker had always told me that if I felt particularly bad I could go to the hospital and speak to the duty psychiatrist. In the past I wouldn't have dreamt of doing that. In the past if I wanted to die, I didn't want to tell anyone. I didn't want to be stopped, but now I had someone else to think of. Ashley loved me and she didn't want me to die. I didn't want to die. So that's what we did, we went to the hospital.

I remember us in the waiting room. Both of us were crying now, sobbing our hearts out and trying to make sense of everything despite the total insanity that I was experiencing. We had to wait for over an hour before I got to see anyone and for the whole time we wept and spoke of how we loved each other and how I was sorry and didn't mean to be like this.

"Ok what has happened tonight?" The psychiatrist asked me.

"Nothing's happened I just feel like I am going to kill myself. I have been thinking of suicide."

"Why? Do you not see a reason to live?"

"Yes, that's why I'm here. I want to die but I want to be with my girlfriend. I have to live for her sake." Ashley sat beside me looking bewildered and hurt; her eyes were red from tears.

"How were you going to do it?"

"I was going to take an overdose of my medication."

"This is the Clomipramine?"

"Yes."

"Is it working?"

"Yes. I used to be obsessed with my skin but now I'm not. I'm just depressed."

"You think of yourself as depressed?"

"Yes."

This was going nowhere. I could have made a tape recorder of my answers. I was getting asked the same old things I always got asked and this guy didn't care that I wanted to die he only cared that I hadn't done anything - I hadn't tried to kill myself - and even those times that I had done it did not really bother these people. Did you have to be climbing the walls before they sat up and took notice?

I'm not sure what I expected them to do for me. I think that perhaps I wanted them to keep me safe from myself and if that meant taking me in to hospital then let it be. I needed looking after. I wanted to be wrapped up in cotton wool and wanted to be told that I didn't have to go to work again, but they sent me home.

"I think the best thing you could do is go home with your girlfriend. Take one extra Olanzapine, but keep safe."

I guess going to the hospital had worked. I suppose by telling Ashley and by going to the hospital and waiting for hours, I had got over that peak. I was all set to do it - ready to take the overdose - but now I had gone past that thought and was on the way to recovery. The thing was that no one was tackling the root cause of this. No one was telling me why I felt like this and no one was making it any better. Ashley had to deal with this and her own mental health was not completely stable. I wondered if one day we would just self-destruct.

We went back to Ashley's mum's house where we were greeted with great support. Ashley's mum probably didn't understand what it was like to be inside my head, no one did, but she did her best to be there, to help, to offer a place to stay and a comfort zone for Ashley.

Ashley was my comfort zone. My relationship with her was always good. We enjoyed being together, we loved each other, we loved our little dog, we loved every moment that we had when it was just us. Trouble was that the world was not just us. There was work, there was family, and there were friends. Ashley got very upset that I was still in contact with Carey, Andie and Phoebe and she was not just thinking of herself she was thinking of me too. These people were leeches. They took from me but did not give anything back and I was still clinging to them, because I was 'too nice' to just say "leave me alone - I have Ashley now." I let those relationships dwindle into nothingness half for Ashley's sake and half for my own. It wasn't easy for me putting my past behind me, I am someone that believes the past is important, but I had Ashley now and I did not need anyone else. That is one of the reasons I decided to write this book, putting everything to bed. The past is just that - it is past.

Choose Life

My life, although with Ashley, was getting hard to live again. It was hard having to go to work. I was getting down like I had before, almost as bad as I had been before meeting Ashley. There wasn't anything particularly wrong with my life except that the depression was back, and I was starting to dread each day and all the time I was not with her. It was a habit I was clinging on to; frightened to be a new person, someone I did not recognise, someone that could be happy.

I hated my job and it was getting harder not to show it. I disappeared for an hour at a time, hiding in the toilets feeling like I was going crazy, feeling like I could not be with any company at all. I would try to do my job but I would despair because it all just seemed so pointless. I would hide in the other warehouse where no one else was working, giving myself jobs that I could do on my own. I took photos of myself with my phone and renamed them 'want to die', 'will I die' and 'Close to death'. I wanted to see if I could see the suicide in my stare. I hated everyone else that worked with me there, not because they were bad people but because they were there, in my face, in my life. I wanted it all to leave me alone. I left work at lunchtime and I had no intention of going back. I left an e-mail for my boss to read.

'I am not coming back today I am very unwell. Take it as holiday - take it as sick I really don't care.'

I rode away from work frightened that I might see someone and they might talk to me. I just wanted to be gone from there, away from all of them. I rode away, pedalling fast so that the air would purify my lungs, finding it hard to breathe, as I no longer wanted to. I wanted to die.

I locked up my bike and went into the off license by the train station and bought a four pack of beer. It still amazed me that I was legally allowed to buy alcohol. Every time I bought some without being asked for identification was a novelty to me. I guess that's because in my mind I am still a child. Maybe that is why I find it so hard, living in an adult world. I left and I went to the train station. I went down the steps and I sat on the bench. There was no one around. I sat there and my thoughts descended further in to darkness and I knew exactly what I was doing. I was going to put an end to all of these thoughts. No more would I have to deal with all the insecurities and hang ups. I was going to jump in front of a high-speed train and be free of all the things my brain subjected me to. No possibility of survival, just a sudden intense pain and then nothing, a mess for the workers to clean up, and a total freeing of my brain. I waited for the next fast train to pass. I looked up at the video screen and it was blank. I waited and then I saw it coming. There were lights in the distance. A train was clattering towards me.

I took a huge swig of beer and I watched it getting closer. Any minute now I would stand up and jump down onto the tracks. Just a little while longer and I wouldn't have to worry about anything ever again. I wouldn't have to worry about work; I wouldn't have to worry about sex; I wouldn't have to worry whether I was being a good boyfriend; I wouldn't have to worry about whether I was pure or not. This would be pure, this last act, the last thing I would ever do.

The train went noisily by me; carriage after carriage and then it was gone. I had sat there and I had watched it

258

and now it was going and I was back to where I had been before, too scared to end my life but too scared to live it. I drank some more beer and put the empty can in the bag. I had another three; I had the chance to get the courage. I would sit here for as long as it took.

Time went by, people came and people got on the next train that stopped at the station. They left and I stayed, drinking beer and watching everything that went on, paranoid that everyone knew what I was doing yet sad that they had no idea. Once their train had left I waited for the next fast train - the next train that would not stop. I wondered if the driver would see me and stop once I was dead. I wondered if people would start complaining about the lateness of the train unaware of the personal tragedy that had caused it. I wondered if they would have any sympathy or whether they would just be annoyed that they were held up on their journey. I wondered if there was any real sympathy for a suicide and whether I was just doomed to be forgotten.

I didn't think about Ashley. If I had thought about her I wouldn't have been

doing this. I really believed that I was alone. No one understood the pain I lived with and therefore no one could help me live. The next fast train was approaching, I had drunk two beers and my brain was fuelled with self-hatred and finality. This was it, this was the end.

...But the train just past and I cursed myself for my indecision and for my cowardice. I sat there and I drunk another beer and I was totally afraid; afraid that I would not have the strength to do this and would have to live, but also afraid that I would and that this really was the end for me. I didn't want this for me. I didn't want to die but I did not want to live in the real world. I was a wreck.

After a while I knew when the next fast train was due. Every time one was due to pass I psyched myself up to make the decision, to make those small movements that would put me on the track in front of the train, in front of my death. ...But I didn't have the guts. Perhaps something was keeping me alive. Perhaps I did think of Ashley somewhere in my foggy thoughts. Perhaps I realised how stupid this was. I had a good life. I had a job, a home and a girl that loved me. I wanted to die but perhaps I just didn't want to die enough to do anything about it. Perhaps you really have to have a reason to kill yourself, and my only reason was that I wanted to be dead. I guess it just wasn't enough.

I was disappointed with myself but it was obvious that I was not going to die today. I had to tell someone what was going on with me. I had to get help and so I went to the mental health clinic to see my social worker. I sat there and I waited for him to come and when he did, I sat in the office and I cried deep sorrowful tears telling him what I had just done. I felt truly sorry for myself and truly sorry that I had even thought of doing this to Ashley. My social worker called her and she came to get me. I could see the hurt behind her eyes although she acted very mature and strong for me. She cradled me in her arms and she took me home. I cried and I told her I was sorry. I didn't really know why this had happened again. I didn't know what triggered me into taking such drastic measures.

Ashley and I had our own world and I wanted to spend all my time there. I wanted to be at home with her just cuddling up with her and our little dog. It was everything else that I wanted to get away from; work, money, mental anguish.

I wanted them to increase my medication but every time I went to see my doctor he just said to keep on doing as I was, but it obviously wasn't working was it? I was back with the Letchworth mental health team now and the doctor there hardly gave me a chance to say what was wrong and how I felt. He just asked the specific questions that they always asked and I gave my short answers. Mere minutes later, the doctor had made his conclusions.

"Ok. Keep on taking the medication, one hundred and fifty milligrams of Clomipramine and ten milligrams of Olanzapine, cut down on the drinking and we will see you in three months."

It was just as well I had a social worker that I could speak with. He was the one and only person that I could tell everything, and being able to say how you are feeling to someone does help. Bottling up all your problems is dangerous because they come out eventually. Leave them in your mind festering, dark and twisted, and they will come out by self-harm or some other break-down. I knew that all too well. I could feel it coming, could feel all those bad thoughts swelling in my head. Then I would cut. I still did it quite often but it was hard to do it with Ashley around. I would have to pretend I was just going to the toilet but I would kneel on the floor and use a broken razor to lash out at my wrist. There were loads of scars now and I was past caring. After the first stinging pain, the cuts stopped hurting and I could do it quicker and harder and then let the blood drip in to the toilet. I liked seeing my arm covered in blood. I liked the way it congealed under my arm. It was my crux, it was my way of dealing with it and it didn't harm anyone, not really.

I realised that if I could change one thing in my life it would be my job - I hated it. I dreaded every single day that I had to go there, and I had to go there for the best part of my life. It wasn't fair that we humans had made life so difficult for ourselves. We had invented money and careers, the whole rat race, and I was forced to be part of it because I was alive. Why wasn't there another choice? Why was it just life or death? If I had another option perhaps I would obsess over that like I obsessed over death, but I knew that I didn't want life, not really.

261

So I got up every day and I kissed Ashley good bye and I went to work and did those stupid tasks for the sake of someone else, for a company I didn't give a shit about just so that I might have a place to rest when I finally got home. It doesn't sound like a good idea does it? Yet every one did it. They just got on with it and they did it, every single day. Why was it so much harder for me to be like them? Ashley also felt like me, she didn't want to do her job either. So I told her to quit. Knowing how awful my job made me feel I could understand why Ashley was miserable and I was earning enough to run the flat. So, because things for her were just getting worse I told her to quit, and she did, and she felt so much better.

For weeks I just got on with this life, going to work, coming home and being with Ashley. The love we had for each other never dwindled, we were as crazy about each other as we had been to begin with but although we had each other, our lives were not heading in a positive direction. Ashley didn't know what she was going to do in the future and I just got on with the job I had knowing that I probably wouldn't want or be offered a promotion. In fact, things at work were getting worse.

My boss gave me a letter that if broken down said "we don't believe you are really ill unless the doctor says you are". They wanted a letter from my doctor to explain what was wrong with me that might mean I had to not be at work. I guess I pushed them over the line when I ran off half way through the day. I guess I had just had too many days off and they were going to try and sack me. I wasn't that bothered though, for I knew that I was truly ill, I knew that I could get a letter that explained things to them. I wasn't faking this. They said they wanted to know so that they could make things easier for me at work, but I knew what they were doing. My boss had always been supportive of me despite all the days off, times I was late and afternoon appointments, but I guessed he was getting pushed by the guys 'up stairs'. I was sure that if they could fire me they would be happy.

When the doctor sent the letter to my bosses they sent a copy to me, and for the first time since being under psychiatric care I had a real diagnosis.

'Mr. Westwood has been with our psychiatric services for ten years. His presentation has been of an emotionally unstable personality disorder with persistent low mood symptoms. Mr. Westwood also suffers from dysmorphophobia and whenever he cannot cope with his stress he has self-harmed. I note that he has managed work quite well for your company for a number of years and I do not think that he has got the sort of disability at the moment that means he will not be able to continue the work he is doing. Mr. Westwood's life is at the moment stable with a stable relationship. A stable job will give him continued stability and structure in his life, which can only benefit him mentally. From time to time, even with all this stability in his life, he will be unable to cope with the stress he perceives and will not be able to cope with his urges to self-harm. During these times he may need to stay off work and to have intensive medical support. His employers will need to be more considerate during these periods and can help him with time off work. Currently with medication and with his stable relationship, Mr. Westwood's mental state is beginning to improve. He still has urges to hurt himself and at times these urges get overwhelming. He also has feelings of a low mood increasing from time to time. With all these difficulties, Mr. Westwood still wants to stay well and make his life worth living for himself. As far as I know, Mr. Westwood wants to continue to work. He has not identified any potential risk factors in his work.'

It was supposed to make my employer more understanding, but it made them want me to go. I guess I wasn't worth the time. I guess I was not so good at my job that they would put up with this head case working for them. I thought I had learnt a lot in my work and was just starting to get good at the tasks I did every day. I was tackling things quite well, but then my boss, Keith called me in to his office.

"Stephen, I have been approached by Tom," Tom being the boss above Keith, "and he is making an offer that if you would like to leave to concentrate on your writing or what ever you might like to do, we would be in a position to offer you a sum of money to go with."

So they wanted to pay me to leave? I couldn't understand why they would be doing that. Then I remembered the letter and the fact that the letter pretty much tells them that they have to let me have time off and I will continue to be unreliable. They couldn't sack me because I was only sick - you can't sack some one for being ill. So they had concocted this devious little scheme.

I said that I had no intention of leaving, which I really didn't. I didn't like working there but I knew my job, it was better the devil you know. I didn't want to have to try and find a new career as this one paid my bills; this one was with the people I had got used to and was friendly with. Why should I want to leave? So I turned his strange offer down and got back to my work.

Days later he called me in again.

"Right, we are having a shuffle about in the warehouse and I have to tell you that your position is no more. You will go back to working with the boys picking and packing."

I was being demoted, being sent back to doing what I did when I first started five years ago.

"I'm afraid we can't rely on you to be here and so we really need to give your position over to someone that has better attendance. Ok? That will start as from now."

He may as well have punched me in the stomach. Everything I had worked for over the last few months was being thrown back in my face and why? It was obvious, they wanted me to leave.

I got up and left the office and headed straight for the toilets. I thought I was going to cry but I didn't, I just stood with my hands clutching the sink and stared at the mirror, scowling into my own eyes. It is so surreal to do that, to look at yourself looking at yourself, it feels like you are being detached from your body. I wished that I could leave my frame, could be away from here. I couldn't go back to do that job, not after I had once been so much better off. I was so upset that they had stopped valuing me, and I valued myself even less.

I left the toilet and went back into the office; I ignored Keith completely and started rummaging around in my stuff to find a Stanley blade. I got one and stormed out, heading back for the toilet, avoiding everyone's eyes lest they talk to me and break my concentration. I locked myself in the cubicle and I did not think, I just did it, I slashed and slashed until my arms were red with blood and covered in long cuts in all different directions. I did it fast and it only took seconds and then I just stood there with my arm dripping blood into the sink, staring at myself again, staring at my blood in the mirror. It was only then that my emotions began to numb and the facts of what all this meant became clear. I wrapped tissue over my wounds like a bandage and pulled down my sleeve. I washed all the blood away and left the toilet. Some one asked if I was all right and I just nodded and kept on walking, heading in to the office to speak with Keith again.

"Keith. Is that offer for a pay off still there?"

"Yes." He didn't seem surprised and was rather calm. "Do you want to speak with Tom?"

"Yeah."

Keith made a phone call and I sat there, my arm stinging with pain as I touched it, pushing the tissue down to soak up the blood before it started running down my hand.

"You can go up to his office now."

I went to Tom's office and I sat down, feeling fragile, feeling broken, so close to tears. I had a figure in my head, an amount of money that I would accept.

"We would be willing to pay you five grand, untaxed."

It was a higher sum than I thought and it would give me five months to find another job, but what other job was going to put up with me? How could I take a new job and have to try and act normal? How could I promise an employer that I was going to be in every day? ...But I accepted the money and I went down stairs to say my good byes.

"Everyone." I called out and Keith was standing behind me with my bag. The small work force that I had got to know and that had become my friends all gathered round realising that something was going on. "I'm leaving," I said, loud enough so that they could all hear. "I'm going now and

I won't be coming back." I felt tears choke in the back of my throat.

They were all puzzled but none of them asked me why they just mumbled their disbelief and each one, in turn, shook my hand and wished me well. Moments later I was riding away for the last time. I felt sad, but I felt that I had done the right thing. They obviously wanted me to leave and I knew from past experience that they could make things harder for me as time went on. So I left with my dignity in tact, if that meant anything, and I felt stabbed in the back, that I had tried so hard for them and this is what I get. By the time I got home I was feeling even worse and Ashley greeted me and I hugged her and I cried. The morning's pain all came crashing down at once. The betrayal, the fear of being without an income, the whole experience just shook me up.

Ashley was not cross with me, she stood by my decision and I knew that I had been given little choice. After a time, Ashley and I discussed the money situation and decided that it was a blessing in disguise. If I wasn't well enough to hold down a job I should be able to get some kind of incapacity benefit. Just because my illness was mental it didn't make it any less real, but even I wondered if I was faking it. Making the government accept my illness seemed to be the next problem to face. Wouldn't they just tell me to 'pull my socks up' and get on with it and what would my family say about it? They all knew my history yet they probably wouldn't be behind my decision to refrain from work. I knew what my mother would say. Every time I had a day off work she had a go at me telling me that they would sack me rather than caring that I was actually too ill to be there. I couldn't tell her because I couldn't cope with the animosity.

I went to the doctor and I went through my history with him. I explained what had happened at the train station and how I just didn't feel that I could work right now. I felt like I was taking a lie detector test, that I was being evaluated to see if I was truly depressed or just trying it on. Despite years of living with this, despite the therapy and the medication it still seemed that no one would perceive me as 'ill'. However, the doctor was very understanding. He signed me off for three months. I knew that wouldn't be enough. My true belief was that I would never be well again.

I tried to think positively about what had happened. I could take some time away from the rat race; I could write and spend time with Ashley and then maybe I wouldn't feel like hurting myself anymore. With a new life away from work, away from having to cope each day in front of all those people, perhaps I could live.

We went out to walk around Hitchin and we bumped into my mother.

"Why aren't you at work?"

"I've got the day off."

"Why? You're not off sick again are you?"

"It's a holiday."

Why did I have to tell her everything I did anyway? Wasn't this my life? We talked for a little while but I felt anxious and sick. I hated lying and hated that I had to lie. I knew what she would be like if I told her I'd lost my job and I didn't want to hear it, I didn't need to be told how awful it was. I knew that it was dysfunctional, but I was dysfunctional, I couldn't cope in the real world. I would tell her at some stage but not right then. Seeing her shook me up, it was a reality check, there were other things, things out side my comfort zone, things besides my happy life with the girl I loved, things that one day I would have to face.

We decided to go on holiday and we had some spare money to play with thanks to losing my job. We decided to get a last minute deal. Turned out 'last minute' was not far from the truth - we booked to go the very next day. It felt quite exciting to do that although I felt a little guilty, thinking that if I was not well enough for work then perhaps I shouldn't be well enough to go on holiday, but it didn't mean that did it? I could lead a fairly normal life - I just couldn't work - not when I had to be around other people. The only job I could really do was writing - working from the seclusion of my own home. I would go on this holiday and maybe, just maybe it would help me to feel better.

We had a good time away in Feurteventura. We went for boat rides and went to a lovely animal park. We were both sick for a day each, but we were spending quality time together and to be on holiday with someone that I loved and who gave me equal love back, was a new experience. We were fine as long as the world left us alone - just us - just Steve and Ashley - that's all I asked for.

Every new experience with Ashley was another memory for us and us alone. This was a new life we were building, living as though there never was a time that we were not together. It felt awful that she had been with another guy and that I had loved in my past. We tried not to think about that. This was a true relationship - a love based on real people for real reasons. On another trip to Great Yarmouth, a place that we had claimed as our own, we got matching tattoos. I would never have thought of doing that with any other girl I had been with. I would never have done it with Carey. I think we just knew that we were going to be together forever, it just seemed obvious. We had a motto 'you and me versus the world', so that's what our tattoos said, written in each other's hand writing on the inside of our arms. That is probably the only tattoo that I haven't regretted for a minute.

As time went on Ashley got a part time job and I got to work on my third novel. I had an idea of a man, obsessed with death that made friends with ghosts. That was the basic premise and soon enough I had all the notes I needed to embark on the new book. I spent hours writing, and I remembered how good writing made me feel, how it actually felt like I was doing something constructive with my life. I didn't care that I wasn't doing a day job because this was my day job. If I were just sitting around the house playing my retro computer games, then maybe I would think I was wasting my life, as it was I was making art, and doing what I always wanted to do. If it weren't for the lack of money I would have been living the dream, but then, if I had more money it would have probably just gone on cider. I had to cut down my drinking and that was very hard for me, though probably for the best.

My mother phoned me one day and my ruse broke down.

"I've just been on the phone with Keith," my old boss. "I wanted to speak to you and he told me that you don't work there any more. What are you playing at?"

"I don't work there anymore. They wanted to get rid of me so I left."

"But you lied to me; you said you were on holiday."

"That's because I knew how you would react."

"Well I was very embarrassed. Why did they want to get rid of you? Because you kept being off sick no doubt. We've tried everything to keep you in that job, I've been to see Keith when you have done things to yourself and he told me they were behind you, what happened?" She was acting exactly as predicted. She didn't care how I felt, only how it affected her.

"They couldn't fire me because I had the doctor's notes so they just made it so bad for me that I would leave on my own accord."

"So what are you going to do now? They were good to you at that job, I felt proud of you that you went to work. It's not easy finding another job you know, especially if you are going to keep being off sick all the time."

"I'm not looking for another job."

"So you're just going to sit at home all day? That's no good for you, you have to get out there and live. You'll just get depressed again if you sit around the house all day."

"I am depressed, that's why I lost my job, that's why I can't work."

"Rubbish. You have to work don't be so stupid..."

She wouldn't let it drop. She made me feel like I was this great failure, that what I was doing was educationally and morally wrong. She kept saying how she had helped me keep that job and that she felt that I should be in work and that she couldn't cope. She wouldn't take any of my explanations and she kept reminding me of all the times I had taken time off and all the good things Keith had once said about me. She just made me feel awful. Once she was off the phone I went in to the bathroom and slashed the hell out of my arms. I knew that I didn't agree with what she was saying but it wasn't nice to hear it. Why couldn't she be supportive and perhaps say "that's a shame how do you feel?" Well it seemed she didn't care how I felt because here I was cutting up my skin because of her, because I was such a disappointment to my family and to the world.

Ashley was a constant support and she hated my mother for the way she had made me feel.

"I try so hard," Ashley said, "to make you feel better and then she comes along and messes it all up in one phone call. You were doing so well."

I was doing better now I wasn't at work. I felt bad that Ashley had to work for I knew that she was not much better at being with people than I was. There was still part of me that felt that a man should provide for his family, but I was providing in a way. By being ill, I was receiving benefits and we worked out our finances and we were no worse off. I was better in health and Ashley didn't mind working at the pizza restaurant part time because she knew it was not permanent. The future could offer much more. Ashley was going to go to college and maybe, just maybe I could get a book published.

One night, after Ashley and I had made love, I lay beside her drifting off to sleep and she whispered, "Marry me."

I think she thought I was asleep. I opened my eyes and turned to look at her, hardly able to keep awake. "You don't mean that," I said.

"Want to bet."

I smiled and closed my eyes again.

"Would you wear white?" I said; sleep starting to creep back over my conscience.

"Probably black," she answered - turns out she wore red.

We spoke about it some more and we decided that there was no point in thinking anything else about it, if we loved each other, if we couldn't imagine a time that we would be apart, we should just do it, we should get married. I didn't actually ask her until Christmas day but we had already started making plans. It took a year to plan, a year of ups and downs. We set the date for next Halloween, a fun time to have it, and forever Halloween would be our anniversary.

When I told my family at Christmas it went down like a lead balloon. They pretended to be happy for us but I knew them well enough to know that they had their doubts. I guess they all thought it was too soon. I guess they didn't realise how happy Ashley made me. If they could see through my eyes, if they could be a fly on the wall, they would know that it was right. Ashley and I had a great relationship. However, my mother, my grandmother and even my sister seemed completely uninterested in it. Perhaps it wasn't exciting to them because I had been married before. Perhaps I was asking too much for them to actually agree with something I was doing for a change.

We heard rumours from one family member to another that things were being said. Things like "this wedding is not going to happen," things like "they won't be able to afford a wedding", and they seemed to delight in the thought that it would all go wrong. Ashley's family was all excited and looking forward to it, my family, excluding my father, was wishing it all to fail. My mother said that she didn't think I was well enough to make such a decision and she put Ashley down as if she wasn't good enough for her son. I resented all of them for the way they were acting and I was getting constant phone calls from my mother trying to run my life for me, still going on about how bad she felt that I had lost my job and that this wedding was happening. My dad was the only person in my family that was happy for me and he was getting very annoyed with the way my mother was acting, as was Ashley's mum. So they wrote her a letter to tell her that she should be happy for us and to stop trying to put a downer on everything. That didn't go down too well.

Writing letters was my mother's favourite trick. By writing a letter she could say exactly what she thought without getting anything said back. I kept getting letters from her with little newspaper clippings about depression and about how being off work was not good for me. Christ why couldn't she let it drop? If I thought that being off work was better for me, why couldn't she believe that? Did she not want me to feel better, to be safe? Perhaps she didn't. Since being with Ashley, I saw a lot less of my mother than I did when I was alone and sick. Perhaps she liked it better when I was ill - then she had someone to hang around with - then she could feel needed as my mother. That's what seemed to be happening and I wrote her a letter myself that said just that; a few home truths.

My mother took the letter as a personal insult and completely ignored what it was actually about. Then, my grandmother got involved saying how badly I was treating my mother and how disgusting the letters were and that they should never have been sent. Never mind all the letters my mother had sent me - never mind all the things she had said to me about losing my job and being with Ashley. We all stopped speaking to each other after that. I worried that it had gone too far, upset that I had hurt my mother's feelings yet completely adamant that the things I had said were true. Neither of us wanted to back down.

The destruction of my family was not complete until my eldest niece announced that she was not going to be our bride's maid after all because she was going on holiday. It had been mentioned tentatively one day while Ashley and I were visiting my sister and we told them how upset we would be if that happened. Then it happened and my sister told me by text.

'Bad news Steve, Amy will be on holiday so won't be going to your wedding. sorry.'

I was furious. We had told them months ago what date we were getting married and that they would need to book the holiday a little earlier or a little later than planned so that Amy could still come to our wedding. Now they were kicking us in the teeth and saying that a holiday was more important to them than us getting married. I was hurt and upset and I sent a text back in the heat of the moment.

'Oh right why don't you all just go on a little picnic and not come to my wedding then'

I didn't get an answer right away but when I did it would put an end to the friendship I had with my brother in-law and would put a crack in the family forever. It was my brother in-law that answered the text.

'After a discussion, Jane and I have decided that none of us are coming to your wedding so don't bother to keep in touch'

Lovely. That was just great. So my sister, my nieces, my mother and my grandmother were all against me. They were all not speaking to me and were all not coming to my wedding. I hadn't felt this bad for weeks. I hadn't cut myself for quite a while, but this was all such a mess in my head that I could not cope with my emotions. When everything is such a mess you need to get some clarity back and there is nothing that clears your mind as much as slashing your wrists. I locked myself in the bathroom and went at it with the razor blade. I was vicious, so much self-hatred, so much inner turmoil, so much anger at how I was being treated, at how Ashley had been treated, and all we had wanted was for people to be happy for us.

Some of my cuts were quite deep so I wrapped toilet paper around my arm and left the bathroom. Ashley knew what I had done; there was no point in hiding it. She didn't even try to stop me anymore because she knew it helped my mind sometimes. Anyway - she couldn't say much about it when she herself turned to that crux occasionally. She knew how it felt to need to do that. The trouble with me though was that I just didn't care how much damage I made. I didn't care if I had to go to hospital and get sewn up. I didn't care if I severed a main vein. I didn't even care if it killed me.

I sat on the sofa with my mind stirring everything around like some bubbling witch's stew. I was breathing heavily, trying to calm myself down and Ashley was there, looking sad and came and knelt beside me to clean my wounds. One of the cuts just wouldn't stop bleeding and although I insisted that it was all right, Ashley was adamant that we should go to the hospital.

Ashley sent an angry text to my sister telling them what I had done because of them and then we went.

I had two male nurses trying to look inside the cut to see how deep it was but they couldn't get the bleeding to stop. They had me sit there with my arm raised holding gauze against the wound and then they would come back to have another look. It wouldn't stop. The men seemed a little incompetent and at a complete loss as to what to do with a cut that wouldn't stop bleeding. At length a different nurse came to have a look and she wiped the wound and looked at it.

"It's fine," she said, "just put some strips to hold it shut."

So that's what they did, I hadn't severed anything important, not this time.

Without the blessing of my family the wedding plans went on. We didn't want a long engagement, we wanted to be married, but the date was set, October the thirty first. This was the wedding I should have had in the first place. What I had with Carey was all her choices, was all hers. Ashley and I were planning this together and every choice was mutual. We chose the music, we chose the venues and we made a list of guests including all my old friends that I had not seen in years. There would be a lot of people that were not there, but that was their loss, we would have a good day anyway. I would have my father and his side of the family, I would have my friends and Ashley's family would all be there, it turned out to be about sixty guests.

I got back in touch with my old friends Rick and Dave and also wrote to Michael. They were happy to hear from me and were positive when I told them I was getting married. I invited them to come round to my house for a stag do. Ashley had a hen night out with her friends and I stayed in with mine. It seemed we were doing everything right, everything we were supposed to do. I got very drunk after taking shots of absinthe and was sick in the sink, but we had a good night catching up with each other.

Ashley slept at her mother's house the night before the wedding and I was alone with my thoughts. Now was the time that I could have been feeling regrets, now was the time it could have all dawned on me and I could see clearly what I was doing, but I had no doubts. I was excited. I had a few drinks and listened to music and when the morning came I calmly got ready without a battle with the mirror.

I was dressed in a black frock coat with lavish gold embroidery over it, a white satin poet's shirt, and black velvet trousers and carried a skull capped walking cane.

This was the Goth wedding I always dreamt of and not once did I doubt it, not once did I think that it wasn't right. I was going to marry the girl that I always should have married, the girl that I loved and the girl that loved me - me, for who I really was, the man I had discovered after the split with Carey, the man that had been through hell to get here, the man I always was.

My father was best man and had in fact proved to be the best man in my life. He picked me up to drive me to Knebworth where the wedding was to take place. I was early and nervous by now that I would not do everything right, nervous as to whether all our hard worked plans would go without a hitch, but never once worried about whether I should be doing this.

The pumpkins were on the tables with their heart shaped holes cut in to them by myself the day before. The reception room had been decorated, the music was playing and all the guests were arriving. This was really happening. After all that planning, after a year of talking about it, it was finally happening. I wondered if I would even have a chance to enjoy the day through all the nerves and excitement, and then, it began. I was standing there by the registrar, and my future wife was walking down the aisle in her red dress, her hair long and black with gold leaves threaded in it, her dress with gold flowers around it, her bouquet of black ostrich feathers and red gerberas. She looked like something out of my most beautiful dreams; she looked like the girl I was going to marry.

They say your wedding day is supposed to be the best day of your life, but I didn't believe in it until that day. There was the romance of the ceremony, making our vows to each other, looking into each other's eyes and seeing true love. There was the emotion of being declared man and wife, so happy that we were, so pleased to have found that truly special person. Then, we walked out of the hall to the wedding song played on guitar by a friend of Ashley's brother. It was all going so well, I was smiling in my heart as well as the grin I had all over my face.

Our car was there waiting for us, a white Beauford with a stream of bubbles flying out from the back. Our names were on an orange number plate at the front. The photographer was organising us, and then we walked out under a shower of confetti with all those people that were there because they cared about us, and we were truly the most important people that day. I didn't think about the people that were not there.

Photographs were taken in the lavish gardens in front of that magnificent stately home. We enjoyed all the posing; we wanted some good pictures of us together. The newspaper reporter turned up to take a picture of the 'Goth' wedding. It was all going so well and I did have time to enjoy it. I kept taking a check of my brain and I realised that I enjoyed every single moment, and I will never forget those moments. We danced the first dance, a song from Labyrinth that had become 'our movie' and 'our song'. We danced with a stream of bubbles dancing with us from the bubble machine. We danced as romance filled our hearts and made us feel warm and safe and so very, very happy. We would never have to be in those dark realms ever again. We had each other forever now. We were safe. Together we would take on the world, together we were perfect.

'Dear diary,

I have been through a lot to get this far in life and everything that has happened has mounted up on top of me like the soil over my casket, but I am not alone anymore. That is the difference. I had been alone for nearly thirty years, and the loneliness really got to me. Alone in a world I want no part of I am close to death, with that special partner

279

in this world I want no part of, I can just about get through the days. I have been depressed for the best part of my life, and I am still depressed now, but now I live; now I am a married man with a possible future, now I choose life.

There are two of me living in this body and one of them wants me dead, one side of me will probably always think about death as a warm electrical blanket wrapped around my soul, but the other me knows that death is just cold. Death might never give me the release I need. I might die and never know one single thing more. I might die and leave my wife distraught and my family with a hole that won't ever be filled. For it doesn't matter what I think about myself, others think differently. I can not understand why

there are people that love me, I can not get in to their heads and hearts and see what they really feel, but if I believe them I need to believe that what they feel for me is love, and that leads to loss.

Not all my family were at my wedding, and a wedding is supposed to bring people together not drive them apart, but that is all done with now. I will never forget that they were not there or the things they said, but people don't always do what you want them to. My sister has spoken to me and put it all behind her, and I have been man enough to do the same. I speak to my mother now and hope that we never have to fall out again, because my family is important to me, because it all hurts. It all adds up, and when I was not speaking to my family I had that hole in my heart. My sister has been ill for years, and a thought occurred to me the other day: With her illness overshadowing my life, making me less important, maybe somewhere in my subconscious I felt that I too had to be ill in order to get any attention. Perhaps my illness had to be worse. Perhaps that is why I embrace my misery and refuse to get better, but I am so much better than I was. I still have to wear make up and I still avoid people and panic if I think they're looking, but

I no longer spend every hour of the day afraid of what I look like. No longer am I shut off from the world.

My family does care, and even if it is just for their sake, I must choose life. Even though each day I feel pain and apathy and sometimes even less than that, I have to go on. Ashley says that her one greatest fear is that one day she will come home and find me dead - that is what I should try to avoid. Forever I said, but I always had a way out. I never said how long forever would be. My forever might be shorter than everyone else' forever. Mine might just be until that inevitable day that I end my life by my own hand and sometimes it really does seem to be inevitable. ...But I mustn't spend all my time looking for a clause in the contract. The world is not always against me; despite the way it tests me on a daily basis. I have Ashley now and it's you and I versus the world remember?

My wish to die might never leave. The jealousy I feel each time I hear of someone's death might always be there. The envy I have for those that successfully kill themselves might play on my mind until the day of my own death. Yet I still do this, I still choose life.

...Because I love Ashley, because we will always be together and always should have been. ...Because I have no real spark to ignite the time bomb I carry around with me, and because for her sake, I hope there never will be, I live.'

S.Westwood Suicide Junkie

Printed in the United Kingdom by
Lightning Source UK Ltd., Milton Keynes
136573UK00001B/15/A